Nutrients for Health

Your Guide to Foods and Nutrients for Your Health and For Overcoming Ailments

The Healthy Food Series

By Rod Stone

I0438800

Copyright Notice

Table of Contents

Introduction

"Let food be thy medicine and medicine be thy food" ~ Hippocrates. Hippocrates is considered one of the most outstanding figures in the history of medicine. He is referred to as the "father of medicine" in recognition of his lasting contributions to the field as the founder of the Hippocratic School of medicine.

"The doctor of the future will give no medicine, but will interest her or his patients in the care of the human frame, in a proper diet, and in the cause and prevention of disease." ~ Thomas Edison. Thomas Edison was an American inventor and businessman. He is the fourth most prolific inventor in history.

"Take care of your body. It's the only place you have to live." ~ Jim Rohn. Jim Rohn has been called America's foremost business philosopher.

"Don't eat anything your great-great grandmother wouldn't recognize as food. There are a great many food-like items in the supermarket your ancestors wouldn't recognize as food...stay away from these." ~ Michael Pollan. Michael Pollan has been writing books and articles about the places where nature and culture intersect: on our plates, in our farms and gardens, and in the built environment.

"Life expectancy would grow by leaps and bounds if green vegetables smelled as good as bacon." ~ Doug Larson. Doug Larson was a newspaper columnist and editor for years and his column was syndicated throughout the nation.

"The best and most efficient pharmacy is within your own system." ~ Robert C. Peale. Robert Peale is an author who wrote *"Live Longer and Better."*

"The best doctor gives the least medicines." ~ Benjamin Franklin. Benjamin Franklin was one of the founding fathers of the United States. He was also a leading author, printer, political theorist, scientist, etc.

Dr. Louis Ignarro, Ph.D. (1998 Nobel Laureate in Medicine) in his book *"Health is Wealth"* stated the following:

"YOU"VE BEEN BRAINWASHED. Along with the rest of us, you have been brought up to believe in a certain set of ideas about wellness and disease—a medical mythology—that our greater scientific understanding shows us is simply not true.

The medical mythology myths are:

1. *Disease is inevitable as the human body ages, and we inexorably progress from a state of health and vitality to one of disease and decrepitude.*
2. *Disease is a separate state than the state of being in health.*
3. *Once you have a disease, you are a fundamentally different being.*

4. Once disease takes hold, it's just a matter of time before it "gets you."

5. The progression (or is it regression?) into more and more severe disease and disability is irreversible.

Healthcare has degenerated in a situation where we wait to get sick, and then hope that a doctor will be able to fix the symptoms without ever having discovered or diagnosed the underlying problem or problems.

Disease is actually nothing more than a set of symptoms...that your body exhibits to let you know it is deficient in certain key nutrients."

The Nutrients for Health provides you with hundreds of foods, nutrients and ingredients for your health along with benefits and other useful information. We also have an illness cross reference to help you to a healthy lifestyle.

Although a food or nutrient may help one person with a particular illness, it does not mean it will help all people. The information we provide are not intended as prescriptions or cures.

MORE FOR YOU

As we do with all of our books we have a website to provide you with more information. Check it out at this   location: http://nutrientsforhealth.healthyfoodseries.com/

To your health!

Rod Stone

Power Foods and Nutrient Information

We all experience disease sometime in our life. Have you ever considered the meaning of disease? "Dis-ease" is a lack of ease. When your body is not experiencing the ease and comfort that it's should experience. When looking at the concept of disease and its meaning you see it's unnatural. It is an organic process that is actually a process that results from deficiency.

We should therefore focus deficiencies that cause dysfunction. This is because every human body requires a certain level of key elements – vitamins, minerals, amino acids, lipids, antioxidants, etc. – to function optimally. A deficiency of these critical elements develops, over time, in a certain type of tissue and a state of dysfunction occurs, or a disease happens.

The great thing about the human body is that to "cure" you just need to provide the body with enough of the elements it needs to restore healthy function. However, the greater the damage, the more time it will take for proper levels of key nutrients to restore optimal health.

Studies have shown that certain nutrients are the most important for optimal health. And there are certain foods that do the best job at providing these nutrients. Thus we have what we call power nutrients and power foods. Those along with other key nutrients are discussed below.

Macronutrients

A macronutrient is the class of chemical compounds or elements humans consume in the largest quantity and which provide the bulk energy. These are carbohydrate, fat and protein.

Carbohydrates:

- Carbohydrates is a macronutrient, like protein and fat.
- Carbohydrates are necessary to your health, because every cell in your body uses them for energy. In fact, your brain can only use carbohydrates for energy.
- Complex carbohydrates are high-fiber foods, which improve your digestion. They help stabilize the blood sugar, keep your energy at an even level, and help you feel satisfied longer after your meal.
- Simple carbohydrates can alter your mood, led to cravings and compulsive eating, cause wide swings in the blood sugar levels, and cause weight gain.
- The closer you get to nature, the closer you get to health. Simple carbohydrates are created in a factory – while complex

carbohydrates are designed by nature.

Some examples of healthy foods containing complex carbohydrates

Apples	Apricots	Artichokes	Asparagus
Broccoli	Brown rice	Brussels sprouts	Buckwheat
Cabbage	Carrots	Cauliflower	Celery
Cucumbers	Dill pickles	Eggplant	Garbanzo
Grapefruit	Kidney beans	Lentils	Lettuce
Navy beans	Oat bran	Oatmeal	Okra
Onions	Oranges	Pears	Pinto beans
Plums	Potatoes	Prunes	Radishes
Soybeans	Spinach	Strawberries	Turnip greens
Water cress	Wild rice	Yams	Yogurt

zucchini

Some examples of foods containing simple carbohydrates

All baked goods made with white flour

Candy

Cake

Corn syrup

Fruit juice

Most packaged cereals

Pasta made with white flour

Soda pop

Fats:

- Fat is a Macronutrient which might be hard to understand why we need fat.
- Fats play a vital role in promoting healthy cell function.
- Vitamins A. D. E. and K are fat-soluble, meaning they can only be digested, absorbed, and transported in conjunction with fats.
- Fats are very confusing to most of us.
- Saturated fats basically come from animals and dairy. (Butter and Lard)
- Monounsaturated fats come from vegetables, poultry and nuts. (Olives, Nuts and Avocadoes)
- Polyunsaturated fats include what we call essential fats, because they must be eaten and are essential to our health as well. Polyunsaturated fat can be found mostly in nuts, seeds, fish, algae, leafy greens and krill.
- Omega –3 and 6 are essential polyunsaturated fats.
- Omega – 3 (DHA, EPA and ALA) come primarily from cold water fish. It is also found in flax, fig and raspberry seeds, but only the ALA which then converts in the human body to form EPA. But DHA only comes from the cold water fish and

also the ALA and EPA is more potent when it comes from the fish.

- Omega – 6 comes from vegetable oils, grain, and arachidonic acid from egg yolks and red meat.
- These essential polyunsaturated fats (Omega – 3 and Omega – 6) makes the cells membrane flexible. This helps them to be more insulin sensitive.
- Omega – 6
    - Causes the blood to be more prone to clot
    - Promote rapid growth of cells
    - Induce smooth muscles cells to contract
    - Bring about an inflammatory response
    - Cause pain
- Omega – 3
    - Blood thinner
    - Slows the growth of cells
    - Relaxes smooth muscle contractions
    - Anti-inflammatory response
    - Relieves pain
    - Replaces and repairs the nerves and brain
- During ancient times (hunter / gather period) the ration of Omega 6 to Omega 3 was 2:1.
- The typical American Diet today is 20-

50:1.
- It is suggested that we be between 2:1 and 6:1.
- The following disease have been associated with too high of a ratio:
    - Depression
    - Memory loss
    - Violence
    - Bi-polar disease
    - Schizophrenia
    - Alzheimer's
    - Multiple sclerosis
    - Parkinson's disease
    - ADD and ADHD
    - Learning Disabilities
    - Behavior Problems

Protein:

- The word Protein originated from the Greek word "Porto's" which means to come first.
- Protein is a Macronutrient, meaning the body needs large amounts.
- Protein is found everywhere in your body. Every single cell, tissue, muscle and bone contains protein
- Proteins function in our body to repair body tissues, muscle mass and provide structure.
- They are components of hormones and the antibodies of the immune system.

- Protein plays a critical role in metabolism.
- The building blocks of protein called amino acids is an essential component of virtually every cell in the body.
- A protein-rich diet helps to maximize fat loss while minimizing loss of lean body mass.
- Protein should come from multiple sources with at least 50% coming from plant sources.
- You should have Protein at every meal.
- Protein requirement is based on amount of lean body mass. The avg. female should have 75-100 grams per day, while the avg. man should have 100-125 grams per day.
- Protein helps you feel fuller for longer.
- Causes less of a rise and fall in blood sugar.

Power nutrients

Power nutrients are the key nutrients that have been shown to provide optimal health. They are:

- Alpha – Lipoic Acid
- Amino Acids
- Antioxidants
- Chromium Picolinate
- Coenzyme Q10
- Essential Fatty Acids (EPA & DHA)

- Glucosamine
- Green Tea
- Pomegranate
- Vitamin D

We also want to include Nitric Oxide (NO), even though it is not a nutrient. It is automatically produced by the human body. However, the body's production of NO decreases with age. But, new research shows how we can stimulate our body to produce what we need for improved health. Dr. Louis Ignarro, Ph.D. won the 1998 Nobel Prize in Medicine for his work on NO and has created a product called Night Works that has been shown to help the body increase NO production. It can be found at my product store at: http://herbal-nutrition.net/rodstone.

Some important functions of NO are:

- Lowers the blood pressure when elevated and protects against hypertension
- Prevents unwanted blood clotting and protects against stroke and heart attach
- Lowers bad cholesterol (LDL) and protects against atherosclerosis, heart disease and stroke
- Protects against vascular complications of diabetes
- Protects against early stages of Alzheimer's disease and dementia
- Protects against gastrointestinal ulcers

- Protects against urinary incontinence in women
- Protects against oxidative stress-mediated tissue injury such as inflammation and arthritis
- Functions as the neurotransmitter that stimulates erectile function in both men and women
- Enhances physical performance, shortens recovery and increases endurance during exercise

Power foods

Power foods are the foods that have been shown to help provide optimal health. We have broken them into super food, heath smart and brain boosters.

Super food:
- Acai
- Almonds
- Blueberry
- Cacao
- Camu – Camu
- Chlorella
- Maca
- Moringa
- Spirulina Algae
- Wheatgrass

Heart smart food:

- Almonds
- Apple
- Avocado
- Beans / legumes
- Black tea
- Cheese
- Corn
- Dark chocolate
- Garlic
- Grapefruit
- Green tea
- Oats
- Olive oil
- Onion
- Orange
- Rice
- Salmon
- Soy
- Spinach
- Tea
- Tomato

Brain Boosters:

- Apple
- Avocado
- Banana
- Barley
- Blueberry
- Dark chocolate

- Grapes
- Green leafy vegetables
- Green tea
- Mackerel
- Olive oil
- Salmon
- Sardines
- Strawberries

Nutrients for a health body

There are many vitamins, minerals and other types of nutrients that can be used to achieve optimized personal nutrition. Use this chart to help you identify vitamins and minerals that you could benefit from or that you may not get enough of in your diet.

Vitamin / Mineral	Major Function	Food Sources
Vitamin A / Beta-carotene	Vision, growth, healthy skin, immune function	Spinach, leafy green vegetables, carrots, cantaloupe, broccoli, apricots, fortified milk and breakfast cereals
Vitamin D	Bone health	Fortified milk, salmon, sardines
Vitamin E	Healthy cell membranes; antioxidant	Vegetable oils, nuts, seeds, fortified cereals
Vitamin K	Blood clotting	Green vegetables, milk, liver
Vitamin B-1 Thiamin	Helps obtain energy from foods; healthy nervous system	Whole and enriched grain products, dried beans, meats
Vitamin B-2 Riboflavin	Helps obtain energy from foods	Milk, mushrooms, spinach, liver, whole grains
Vitamin B-3 Niacin	Helps obtain energy from foods	Mushrooms, bran, fish, chicken, beef, liver, peanuts, enriched grains
Vitamin B-6	Helps body to process proteins; healthy nervous system	Meats, fish, poultry, spinach, broccoli, bananas, sunflower seeds

Folic Acid	Protects genetic material and prevents certain birth defects	Green leafy vegetables, oranges, organ meats
Vitamin B-12	Healthy nervous system	Animal foods (not naturally in plants) fortified foods
Vitamin C	Healthy connective tissue; antioxidant	Citrus fruits, strawberries, green leafy vegetables, peppers, tomatoes
Potassium	Healthy nervous system	Spinach, squash, bananas, oranges, tomatoes, melons, dried beans, milk whole grains
Calcium	Healthy nervous system; healthy bones and teeth	Milk, yogurt, cottage cheese, tofu, leafy vegetables and some fortified foods
Copper	Growth, helps prevent anemia	Liver, beans, nuts, whole grains
Iron	Prevent anemia, healthy immune system	Meats, seafood, whole grains, broccoli, peas, bran
Magnesium	Bone strength, nerve and heart function	Wheat bran, green vegetables, nuts, chocolate, beans
Selenium	Antioxidant	Meats, eggs, fish, whole grains

Zinc	Growth, immunity, development	Seafood, meats, greens, whole grains

Beneficial Foods, Nutrients, Ingredients

Our title indicates foods, nutrients and ingredients. This is because of the way of our life. We no longer consume our foods shortly after we or our neighbors harvest them. We also eat much more processed foods than we should. We therefore need to supplement to get the proper nutrients from our food. We also need to look for the proper ingredients in processed foods.

We do not recommend having processed foods. However, we know people. Therefore, when having processed foods you will find that when looking at the ingredients, you will find the less the better! If you see too many names you don't know then avoid!!!

By feeding your body the right blend of key nutritional supplements, you will increase your odds of avoiding acute and chronic health conditions.

In 1988, the U.S, Surgeon General concluded that 15 out of 21 deaths involved nutritional deficiencies.

Every human being, in his or her natural state of being, is a fully holistic entity operating with optimal functionality. It can perform these functions with incredible ease, provided it receives enough of three key elements it requires: proper nutrition, proper exercise, and proper rest. In the following pages we will discuss what you require for proper nutrition.

4D Glucohydrolase:

- Originates from barley
- Is an enzyme
- Shows inhibition of cancer cells in animal studies

Acacia:

- Gum from the Acacia tree.
- Dissolves rapidly in water.
- Retards sugar from crystalizing.
- Used as a thickener for candy and gum.
- Prevents chemical break down in foods.
- Gives form and shape to tablets.
- Used for dysentery & diarrhea.

Acai:

- **Is considered a super food.**
- The acai berry is the fruit of the Acai Palm tree which grows in the flood plains of the Aazon in Brazil.
- Berries contain high concentration of beneficial anthocyanins.
- Supports healthy aging.
- Rich in dietary fiber.

- Abundance of essential fatty acids
- Almost perfect essential amino acid complex.

Acerola Extract:

- From the Acerola cherry.
- Excellent source of Vitamin C.
- Usually combined with rose hips.
- Anti-infective and stress reduction properties.

Alfalfa Extract / Leaves:

- King of restorative, nourishing herbs.
- Roots of plant are very deep which enables it to reach minerals other plants cannot.
- Great for all chronic and acute digestive problems.
- Excellent for arthritic and rheumatoid conditions as well as bursitis and gout.
- Useful in alleviating allergies.
- Helps anemia.
- Blood purifier.
- Decreases morning sickness.
- Diminishes nausea.
- Helps control diabetes.
- Aids the pituitary gland.
- Promotes healthy teeth.
- May help improve halitosis.
- Good for ulcers.

Alliin:

- Sulfur compound that kills bacteria and fungi.
- Active ingredient in garlic.
- Garlic is reported to have cancer preventing, antimicrobial, antibiotic, anti-hypertension, hypoglycemic, and cholesterol-lowering properties.
- Vegetables containing Alliin are known to reduce the risk of stomach cancer.
- Used separately to insure the production of allicin.
- Useful in diminishing the aroma associated with raw garlic.
- May help with parasites and fungal infections according to some studies.
- Garlic is most noted for its promotion of cardiovascular health.
- It is known to help with respiratory infections.
- Good for Legionnaire's Disease.

Allspice:

- Found to have anti-inflammatory, *rubefacient* (warming and soothing), carminative and anti-flatulent properties.
- Useful in gum and dental treatment.
- Good amount of minerals like potassium.
- Good amounts of vitamin A, C, etc.

Almonds:

- **Almonds are a Superfood.**
- **Heart smart food.**
- Seems to have protective properties against heart disease and cancer.
- Aids in bone health and reproductive health.
- Excellent source of vitamin E.
- Cholesterol free.
- Major source of antioxidant *tocopherols*.
- Good source of folic acid, protein, fiber, iron, zinc, and copper.
- Nutritional Facts:
  - Serving Size – 1 oz
  - Calories –163
  - Dietary Fiber – 3.5g
  - Protein – 6g

Aloe Vera Concentrate / leaf:

- Botanical purgative which stimulates the flow and discharge of bile into the small intestine.
- Assists the peristaltic action in the intestinal tract.
- Soothing and healing lubricant for both internal and external use.
- Antibacterial and antifungal properties.
- Helps heal ulcers.
- Has helped clear up acne.
- Wonderful for burns.

- Helps many kinds of skin diseases, i.e. dandruff, dermatitis.
- Helpful in AIDS because of its cleansing and the carrisyn in aloe may work like AZT without the side effects.
- Boosts immune system.

Alpha Lipoic Acid:

- **Is considered a Power Nutrient**.
- Also known as thioctic acid, lipoic acid, lipoate, and dihydrolipoic acid.
- Involved in the conversion of carbohydrates to energy.
- Helps improve blood sugar metabolism and insulin sensitivity.
- Antioxidant nutrient that protects peripheral nerves.
- Reduces neuropathic insufficiency.
- Improves cardiac autonomic neuropathy.
- Prevents free radical damage to eyes.
- Tends to boost glutathione, an antioxidant.
- Works well with other antioxidants such as Vitamin C & E making them more useful.
- Good for people with diabetes especially where there has been nerve damage.
- Slows pre-maturing of skin damage and wrinkling.
- The only known antioxidant soluble in both water and fat, thus can move into all

parts of the cell to neutralize free radicals.
- Studies have found this helpful in people with chronic fatigue syndrome.
- In Germany it is approved in the treatment of diabetic neuropathy.
- Exercise performance aid.
- Reduces the effects of aging.
- Helps with diabetes by improving glucose uptake in insulin-resistant cells.
- Relieves several components of metabolic syndrome by reducing blood pressure and insulin resistance.
- Improve cholesterol and triglyceride levels.
- Helps control weight.
- Effective on cognitive function and brain health.
- Increase antioxidant enzymes in the eye to protect against oxidative damage and curbing cataract.

Amino Acids:

- **Is considered a Power Nutrient**.
- The basic building blocks of all proteins.
- Some can be made by biological processes; some must be provided through diet or supplementation.
- Essential amino acids must be obtained from food. These include lysine, phenylalanine, tryptophan, arginine, and histidine.

- Non-essential amino acids include alanine, asparagine, aspartate, cysteine, glutamine, glycine, and proline.

Amla Extract, Dried (Phyllanthus Emblica):

- Berry from India containing eight times more Vitamin C than lemons.
- Helpful for anemia and diseases that waste and debilitate.
- One of the most used and effective tonic in Ayurvedic medicine.
- Good for convalescence.
- Has laxative, nutritive and rejuvenating qualities.

Anchovy:

- Found in the coldest waters.
- Known to have one of the highest levels of EPA and DHA.
- Considered to be very ecology safe.

Anise seed:

- Anise spice contains antioxidant which are disease preventing and health promotions.
- Anise seeds are an excellent source of many essential B-complex vitamins.
- Great source of minerals like iron, zinc

and potassium. Potassium helps control heart rate and blood pressure.
- Contains good amounts of vitamin A and C.

Antioxidants:

- **Is considered a Power Nutrient**.
- Antioxidants are molecules that pair their own electrons with "free radicals" neutralizing them.
- Antioxidants are considered possible preventive agents for aging, cancer, diabetes, cardiovascular dysfunction and Alzheimer's disease.
- Antioxidants increase the effectiveness of nitric oxide, which dilates blood vessels, contributes to healthy endothelium which helps to prevent cardiovascular dysfunction.
- Antioxidants are abundant in foods such as blueberries, acai berries, apples, pomegranates, strawberries, cherries, plums, sweet potatoes, carrots, pecans and green tea.

Apple:

- Source of major antioxidant *flavonoids*.
- **Heart smart food**.
- **Brain booster**.
- Lowers cholesterol in the blood.

- Contains flavonoids to help cut heart risk.
- Excellent source of soluble fiber.
- Good source of vitamin C and B-complex.
- Prevents some cancers.
- Helps prevent tooth decay by clearing away food particles.
- This source of soluble fiber helps with cholesterol.
- Nutritional Facts:
  - Serving Size – 8 oz
  - Calories –130
  - Fat – 0
  - Dietary Fiber – 5g
  - Sugars – 25g
  - Protein – 1g

Apple Cider Vinegar:

- Has been used to aid in the breaking up of bronchial and sinus congestion.
- Also used as a flavor enhancer and preservative.
- Aids in the digestion of heavy foods, especially protein.
- Great source of potassium.
- Excellent blood cleanser.

Apple Pectin:

- Anti-diuretic.
- Lowers chance of cancer.
- Helps to prevent gallstone.

- Useful for balancing acid I alkaline levels.
- Pectin slows the absorption of food allowing the removal of unwanted metals and toxins.
- Lowers cholesterol and reduces occurrence of heart disease.
- Helps regulate blood sugar levels in diabetics.

Apricots:

- Good source of vitamin A, and C.
- Comes with some important health promoting flavonoids.

Arabinogalactan:

- A dietary fiber from the Western Larch tree.
- Tends to be a food for beneficial bacteria.
- Powerful immune booster.
- Good source of fiber.
- Helps relieve constipation.

Argine:

- **Is an amino acid and is considered a Power Nutrient**.
- Is an amino acid that our body can produce but not at sufficient levels to get it's most dramatic benefits. When oral

ingestion takes place the following benefits are seen:

- It plays an important role in the healing of wounds, removing ammonia from the body, supporting the immune function, and the release of hormones.
- It is the sole precursor to the synthesis of nitric oxide.
- The release of the most important anti-aging hormones.
- Improved immune function.
- Reduced healing time for injuries, particularly bones.
- Reduced risk of heart disease.
- Increased muscle mass.
- Reduced body fat.
- Improved insulin sensitivity.
- Decreased blood pressure.
- Alleviation of male infertility by improving sperm production.
- Increased circulation throughout the body.
- Recommended supplementation of 5,000 to 8,000 mg daily for optimal cardiovascular benefits.

Artichoke:

- Rich source of dietary fiber.
- Overall cholesterol reduction.
- Good source of folic acid, Vitamin C, B-complex.

Arugula:

- Good source of phytochemical which have been shown to benefit against various cancers.
- Good source of vitamin A, B-complex, vitamin C, vitamin K, etc.

Ascorbic Acid (Vitamin C):

- Greatly enhances immunity as well as adrenal gland function.
- Aids tissue growth and repair.
- Good for bones.
- Reduces capillary fragility and enhances iron uptake.
- Prevents hemorrhaging.
- Maintains collagen formation in connective tissue.
- Helpful in replenishing the power of Vitamin E after it neutralizes a free radical.
- Is a water soluble antioxidant.
- Reduces effects of allergy producing substances.
- Fights cancer.
- Optimal level of Vitamin C is approximately 1200 to 2000 mg. daily while the RDA is only 60 mg.
- Note: It would take the consumption of 18 oranges, 17 kiwi fruit, or 160 apples to receive this level of Vitamin C.

Ashwagandha Extract (Root), Dried:

- Used in Ayurvedic Medicine.
- Has a sedative effect.
- Affects the nervous and reproduction system.
- Used medically for weakness and failure to thrive syndromes in children.
- Can help with impotence and infertility.
- May help with joint pain.
- Been used for people with multiple sclerosis.

Asparagus:

- Used in treatment of irritable bowel syndrome.
- Good source of antioxidants protect from cancers, neuro-degenerative diseases and viral infections.
- Rich in vitamin C, vitamin A, vitamin E, and vitamin K.
- Seems to help with neuronal damage in the brain and thus helps Alzheimer's disease.
- Nutritional Facts:
    - Serving Size – 3.3 oz.
    - Calories – 20
    - Fat – 0g
    - Dietary Fiber – 2 g
    - Sugars – 2 g
    - Protein – 2 g

Aspartic Acid:

- **Is an amino acid and is considered a Power Nutrient**.
- Helps to increase stamina.
- Good for fatigue.
- Plays a vital role in metabolism.
- Helps to get rid of harmful ammonia in the liver.
- Protects the nervous system.

Astragalus (Root):

- Powerfully increases metabolic rate and increases energy.
- Protects immune system.
- Helps adrenal glands.
- Is diuretic and promotes healing.
- Legendary aphrodisiac.
- Chinese studies show that it helps with cancer by increasing killer cells (LAK).
- Used for diabetes.
- Shown in Chinese studies to reduce and shorten colds.
- Aids by stimulating activity of T-helper cells without activating T-suppressor cells.
- Helps offset immune damage from numerous drugs.
- **Caution for people taking beta blocks and Warfarin after heart attacks. Should not be used.
- **Caution should be used with people on immunosuppressive treatment and people

who have had transplants.

Avocado:
- **Heart smart food**.
- **Brain booster**.
- Major source of antioxidant *tocopherols*.
- Helps control cholesterol.
- Very good source of soluble and insoluble dietary fiber.
- Good source of vitamin A, E, and K.
- Helps prevent some cancers.
- Nutritional Facts:
  - Serving Size – 1.1 oz
  - Calories –50
  - Fat – 4.5g
  - Dietary Fiber – 1g
  - Sugars – 0g
  - Protein – 1g

Banana:
- **Brain booster**.
- Have beneficial nutrients as well as high potassium content.
- Also contain a healthy dose of vitamin B_6.
- Moderate source of vitamin C.
- Good amount of potassium.
- Controls blood pressure.
- Calms nervous system.
- Helps calm intestinal disorders.
- Lowers risk of strokes.
- **Nutritional Facts:**

- Serving Size – 4.5 oz
- Calories –110
- Fat – 0g
- Dietary Fiber – 3g
- Sugars – 19g
- Protein – 1g

Barberry (Root):

- Benefits the Liver.
- Improves the absorption of minerals.
- Promotes weight loss.
- Cleanses the blood.
- Treats high blood pressure, thick poorly circulating blood, and weak blood vessels.
- Alleviates flatulence and indigestion in general.

Barley:

- **Brain booster**.
- Nutritional Facts:
  - Serving Size – 100 g
  - Calories –123
  - Dietary Fiber – 3.8g
  - Protein – 2.2g

Basil herb:

- Basil leaves contain many notable plants derived chemical compounds that are known to have disease preventing and health promoting properties.
- Essential oils to have anti-inflammatory

and anti-bacterial properties.
- High levels of vitamin A which protect from lung and oral cavity cancers.
- Zea-xanthin which protect from age-related macular disease.
- Vitamin K which strengthens bones.
- Good amount of potassium and other minerals which help control heart rate and blood pressure.

Bay leaf:

- Bay leaf was highly praised by the Greeks and the Romans, who believed that the herb symbolizes wisdom, peace, and protection.
- It has many volatile active components that are known to have antiseptic, anti-oxidant, digestive, and thought to have anti-cancer properties.
- Rich in vitamins A and C.
- Good source of folic acid and B-complex.
- Good source of minerals like potassium which helps control heart rate and blood pressure.

Beans:

- **Heart smart food**.
- Beans were an important source of protein throughout Old and New World history, and still are today.

- One cup of beans provide between 9 – 13 grams of fiber.
- Eating 1 ½ cups of beans daily provides enough soluble fiber to lower cholesterol levels.
- Beans and legumes are a great source of protein. The amount of protein varies greatly from the type of bean. Most means run around 12 – 16 grams of protein per cup. However, soy is over 28 grams and Falafel is on 2.3.
- Rich in folic acid which helps prevent buildup of homocyseine.
- They lower the risk of developing diabetes and cardiovascular disease.
- Help balance blood sugar and lower cholesterol.
- Help with weight loss / management.
- Bean comparison chart next page:

Bean comparison (1 cup)

Bean type	Calories	Carbs	Protein	Fiber	Fat
Black	227	40.8g	15.2g	15g	0.4g
Red	225	40.3g	15.3g	13.1g	.88g
Pinto	245	44.8g	15.4g	15.4g	1.2g
Great Northern	209	37.3g	14.7g	12.4g	0.9g
Lima	216	39.3g	14.7t	13.2g	0.8g
Navy	255	47.5g	15g	19.1g	1.1g
Fava	187	33.5h	12.9g	9.2g	0.7g
Mung	212	38.8g	14.2g	15.4g	0.8g
Black-eyed Peas	220	32g	16g	8g	1g
Garbanzo	269	44.9g	14.5g	12.5g	4.3g
Lentils	230	40g	18g	16g	1g
Soy	254	20g	22.2g	7.6g	11.5g

Bee Pollen:

- Contains many nutrients, i.e. Vitamin B complex, Vitamin C, amino acids, carotene, fatty acids, enzymes, magnesium, iron, copper, calcium, potassium, manganese, and sodium.
- Contains up to 35% protein.
- Antimicrobial effect.
- Slows aging process.

- Good energy food.
- Helps alleviate allergy symptoms.
- Enhance s physical stamina

Beeswax:

- Substance useful for its properties as a carrier for other ingredients, both internally and externally.

Beet:

- Lowers chance of developing heart disease.
- Beet greens are excellent source of vitamin C, vitamin A and other antioxidants.
- Rich in B-complex.
- Cleanses digestive system by bulking waste.
- Sweeps sides of intestines to remove buildup.
- Aids in regulation of bowel movements.
- Useful in alleviating constipation.

Bell Pepper:

- Contains compound capsaicin, which help with anti-diabetic, anti-carcinogenic, etc.
- Rich source of vitamin C and good levels of vitamin A and B-complex.

Berries:

- Source of major antioxidant *anthocyans.*

Beta Carotene (Vitamin A):

- **Is an antioxidant which is considered a Power Nutrient.**
- Slows aging.
- Enhances immunity by protecting mucous membranes.
- Prevents night blindness and other eye problems.
- Great for skin disorders.
- Utilizes protein.
- Key in formulation of bones and teeth.
- Enhances growth and repair of body
- tissue.
- Protects against cancer.
- Protects against infections.

Betaine Hydrochloride (HCL):

- From beet leaves.
- High in hydrochloric acid
- Has good digestive values

Bilberry Extract, Dried (Fruit):

- Helps retard night blindness.
- Anti-carcinogenic.
- Anti-inflammatory.

- Helps with varicose veins.
- Helps with diabetes mellitus (degeneration of the retina).
- Gives strength and support to collagen structure.

Biotin (vitamin H):

- Good for cell growth and fatty acid production.
- Helps in metabolism of carbohydrates, fats, proteins, and the B complex vitamins.
- Important to healthy bone marrow and nerve tissue.
- Stimulates sweat glands and normal skin and hair.
- Is coenzyme in DNA process of cell division and replication.
- Essential to embryonic and fetal development and prevention of mental retardation.
- Is a carbon carrier, brain food and increases energy.

Black Cohosh Extract, Dried:

- Induces labor.
- Good for morning sickness.
- Anti-inflammatory.
- Antispasmodic.

- Good for anorexia.
- Helps reduce anxiety.
- Relieves coughing.
- Delays degeneration of the retina.
- Relieves fibrositis, headaches, hot flashes, hysteria, myalgia, PMS, arthritis, & uterine cramps.
- Lowers blood pressure and cholesterol.

Black Pepper:

- Peppers have been in use since ancient times for its anti-inflammatory, carminative, anti-flatulent properties.
- Composed of health benefiting essential oils. Can increase absorption of other nutrients.
- Contain good amount of minerals like potassium, etc. Helps control heart rate and blood pressure. Essential for cellular respiration and blood cell production.
- Good source of antioxidants such as vitamin A and C.
- Helps nutrients become more bio available by increasing blood flow to the intestinal tract , by increasing emulsifying content of the stomach, and by increasing the active nutrient transport

Black Tea:

- **Heart smart food**.
- Made from the same leaves as green tea.

- Allowed to ferment and age longer than green tea.
- The fermentation process gives a deeper richer flavor but may destroy some of the active and/or beneficial components.
- Contains more caffeine than Green Tea.
- Helps lower cholesterol.

Black Walnut (Leaf):

- Using the leaf as a tea has been useful in lowering blood sugar, cleansing the blood, and eliminating intestinal parasites.
- In tea form useful as an astringent.
- The leaves seem to have an antibiotic element.
- The bark as well as the leaves can be useful in the treatment of skin troubles such as herpes, eczema, or indolent ulcers.
- Works well on diarrhea, constipation, and dysentery.
- Acts as an antifungal and may help in yeast infection.
- Useful in de-worming and eliminating parasites.
- Helps in toning the GI tract.
- Helpful in balancing the intestinal flora.
- Useful in helping with the absorption of oil-soluble vitamins including Vitamin
- B_{12} in association with ileocecal inflammations. The ileocecal valve is located in the digestive tract between the

small and large intestine.

Blonde Psyllium (Seed Husks):

- Fiber which cleans the intestines by absorbing water and expanding many times in size.
- Softens stools and helps body avoid colitis and constipation.

Blueberry:

- **Are a super fruit.**
- **Brain booster**.
- One of the richest sources of antioxidants, and anthocyanin.
- Good source of potassium, folic acid, iron, and Vitamins A & C.
- Contains proanthocyanidins, which can keep e-coli bacteria from harming the urinary track.
- Contains condensed tannins that fight urinary tract infections.
- Appears to slow macular degeneration and improve night vision.
- Studies show promise in helping memory and motor coordination.
- Slows aging and may reduce cancer.

Borage (starflower) herb:

- Very popular herb in Mediterranean countries.

- Contain omega-6 fatty acid gamma-linolenic acid (GLA) that plays vital role in restoration of joint health, immunity and healthy skin.
- High levels of vitamins A and C. Vitamin A protects from lung and oral cavity cancers.
- Good amounts of minerals like iron which determines the oxygen-carrying capacity of blood.

Boswellia Extract, Dried (Boswellia Serrato) (Gum):

- Found to be antifungal, antibacterial, analgesic, sedative, and a powerful anti-inflammatory.
- Tree found in some parts of India.
- Helps with rheumatic conditions.

Broccoli:

- Source of major antioxidant *indoles*.
- Brightens eyes. May fight oxidants and chemicals that cause eye deterioration.
- Has a healthy amount of vitamin C and folic acid.
- Softens rough skin caused by Vitamin A and pantothenic acid.
- Sprouts contain 20 times more Sulforaphane glucosinolate (SGS) than mature broccoli.
- One ounce of broccoli sprouts is the

equivalent of 3.5 cups of mature broccoli.
- High levels of isothiocyanates, a protective chemical, can be found in broccoli sprouts.
- Sulforaphane glucosinolate (SGS) a specific isothiocyanate and powerful phytochemical found in broccoli sprouts can protect against cancer, especially; breast, prostate, colon, urinary bladder and pancreatic.
- High source of sulfur, iron and B vitamins.
- Rich in chlorophyll.
- A natural diuretic
- Nutritional Facts:
    - Serving Size – 5.3 oz.
    - Calories – 45
    - Fat – 0 g
    - Dietary Fiber – 3 g
    - Sugars – 2 g
    - Protein – 4 g

Bromelain:

- Bromelain is an extract derived from pineapples.
- Destroys worms.
- Used in anti-inflammatory medications.
- Works as a blood thinner.
- Reduces swelling and pain.
- Acts as an aid to digestion.

- Reduces symptoms of gout.
- Alleviates bronchitis, sinusitis and respiratory allergies.
- Useful in relieving symptoms of carpal tunnel syndrome.

Brussels sprouts:

- Source of major antioxidant *indoles* and other antioxidants which offer protection from prostate, colon, and endometrial cancers.
- Excellent source of vitamin C, K and B-complex.
- Shown to help with long and oral cavity cancers.
- Also limits neuronal damage in the brain.

Buchu Extract, Short Dried (Leaves):

- Originates from South Africa.
- Good for digestion - gas, bloating.
- Is an excellent diuretic and is used for all acute and chronic urinary
- Fights inflammation of mucous membranes in sinuses due to colds / allergies.
- Aids in controlling diabetes / hypoglycemia.

Buckwheat:

- Rich source of soluble and insoluble fiber.
- Ok source of protein.
- Gluten-free.
- Contains several polyphenolic like rutin, which may offer a cure in hemorrhoids and clotting disorders.
- Good amounts of B-complex.
- Good concentration of minerals that relaxes blood vessels leading to brain and found to have curative effects on depression and headache.
- Nutritional Facts:
  - Serving Size – 100 g
  - Calories –340
  - Dietary Fiber – 10.0 g
  - Protein – 13.2 g

Burdock root:

- Good source of various polysaccharides which act as prebiotic and helps reduce blood-sugar level, weight and cholesterol levels.
- Good amount of potassium to help control heart rate and blood pressure.
- Contains many vital vitamins like C and E.

Butternut squash:

- Good source of vitamin A and B-complex.
- Benefits heart health.
- Eye site
- Protects against lung and oral cavity cancers.

Brazil nuts:

- Excellent source of mono-unsaturated fatty acids help prevent coronary artery disease and strokes.
- Good source of vitamin E.
- High levels of selenium which help prevent coronary artery disease, liver cirrhosis and cancers.
- Gluten free.
- Excellent source of B-complex

Cabbage:

- Storehouse of phyto-chemical which help protect against breast, colon, and prostate cancers and help control cholesterol levels.
- May reduce risk of cataracts.
- May reduce risk of heart disease, and stroke.
- Good source of Vitamin B, C, K and folate.
- Useful for colds.
- Excellent for ulcers and digestive health.
- Nutritional Facts:
    - Serving Size – 3.0oz.
    - Calories – 25
    - Fat – 0 g
    - Dietary Fiber – 2 g
    - Sugars – 3g
    - Protein – 1 g

Cacao Extract, Dried, (Seeds):

- **Is considered a super food.**
- Theobroma cacao is a small evergreen tree native of Central and South America. Its seeds are used to make cocoa powder and chocolate.
- Increases blood flow to the brain and enhances brain function.
- #1 source of magnesium of any food. Helps balance brain chemistry, builds strong bones, regulates heartbeat and blood pressures, helps prevent constipation and eases minor menstrual cramps.
- Raises level of serotonin in the brain; thus acts to regulate mood, help with PMS discomfort, and promote a sense of well-being.
- Stimulate the secretion of endorphins, producing a pleasurable sensation similar to the "runner's high."
- High in sulfur; which builds strong nails and hair, promotes beautiful skin, detoxifies the liver, and supports healthy pancreas.
- Used as a diuretic.
- Known to dilate blood vessels.
- Works on the nervous system and brain to feel better emotionally.
- Is a mild stimulant.

Caffeine:

- Stimulating ingredient.
- Enhances fat oxidation by increasing circulating fatty acids.

Calcium:

- Maintains regular heart-beat.
- Instrumental in blood clotting and balancing acid /alkali in blood.
- Important in muscle growth and contraction.
- Prevents cramps.
- Critical in the formation of strong bones, teeth.
- Affects sleep patterns and the transmission of nerve impulses.
- Contributes to the permeability of cell membranes.

Cambogia Extract, Dried Garcinia (Fruit):

- From type of Garcinia tree native to Asia.
- Decreases appetite thus helping weight loss.
- Stops synthesis of fat.
- Balances sugar metabolism in diabetes.

Camu – Camu:

- **Is considered a super food**.
- Bush that grows in the black water rivers of the South American Amazon rainforest.
- The berries contain the highest amount of vitamin C of any botanical source.
- Berries also contain beneficial phytochemicals.
- Regulates soreness considerably.
- Supports healthy respiratory function.
- Maintains healthy skin, hair and nails.
- Helps support vibrant eyesight.
- Strengthens tendons and ligaments.
- Helps to keep organs such as the eyes, brain, heart, skin and liver in good working condition.

Canola

- Oil lower in saturated fat than others more commonly used.
- Comes from rapeseed plant, a member of the cabbage family and considered to be a weed.

Cantaloupe:

- Excellent source of vitamin A.
- Good source of B-complex and vitamin C.
- Helps in prevention of some cancers.

- Offers protection against stroke and heart diseases.
- **Nutritional Facts:**
    - Serving Size – 4.8 oz.
    - Calories –50
    - Fat – 0g
    - Dietary Fiber – 1g
    - Sugars – 11g
    - Protein – 1g

Capers:

- High in flavonoids which has anti-bacterial, anti-carcinogenic, analgesic, and anti-inflammatory properties.
- Inhibits platelet clump formation in blood vessels.
- Healthy levels of vitamin A and K.
- Good amounts of minerals like calcium and iron.

Caraway:

- Rich in dietary fiber.
- Contain several health benefiting essential oils.
- Has several health benefiting flavonoid antioxidants to protect from cancers, infection, aging and degenerative neurological diseases.
- Excellent source of minerals like iron, cooper, potassium and selenium. Helps in production of red blood cells. Helps with digestion. Helps to control heart rate and

blood pressure.
- Good source of vitamin A, C and B-complex.

Cardamom Seed:

- Good source of minerals like potassium. Helps control heart rate and blood pressure.
- Excellent source of iron and manganese.
- Alleviates pain.

Carnitine:

- **Is an amino acid and is considered a Power Nutrient**.
- Is biosynthesized from the amino acids lysine and methionine, primarily in the liver and kidneys.
- Carnitine concentrations diminish with aging which affect the bones.
- Carnitine also produces substantial antioxidant action in the body, providing a protective effect for cell membranes, particularly in the heart muscle.
- Recommended supplementation of 1,000 to 2,000 mg daily for metabolic support.

Carotene, (Vitamin A):

- Antioxidant.
- Slows aging.
- Enhances immunity by protecting mucous membranes.
- Prevents night blindness and other eye problems.
- Great for skin disorders.
- Utilizes protein.
- Key in formulation of bones and teeth.
- Enhances growth and repair of body tissue.

Carrot:

- Source of major antioxidant *carotenoids*.
- Rich source of beta-carotene.
- Good source of vitamin A, C and B-complex.
- Fights cancer.
- Helps ear problems.
- Skin problems.
- Anti-inflammatory for mucous membranes.
- Increases milk supply for nursing mothers.
- Helps regulate hormones.
- Aids in constipation.
- Calcium metabolism strengthens connective tissue.
  - Nutritional Facts:
    - Serving Size – 2.8 oz.

- Calories – 30
- Fat – 0 g
- Dietary Fiber – 2 g
- Sugars – 5 g
- Protein – 1 g

Cashew nut:

- Rich in monounsaturated-fatty acids which help to prevent coronary artery disease and strokes.
- Rich source of essential minerals. A handful a day will provide enough to prevent deficiency diseases.
- Rich in many essential vitamins which are essential for metabolism of protein, fat and carbohydrates at cellular levels.
- Helps prevent age-related macular degeneration.
- Nutritional Facts:
  - Serving Size – 1 oz.
  - Calories –157
  - Dietary Fiber – 0.9 g
  - Protein – 5 g

Castor Oil (Ricinus Communis) (Seed):

- A colorless or yellowish oil.
- Useful as a cathartic or lubricant, etc.
- Can be used for all liver diseases including

hepatitis and gallstones.
- Used for skin diseases, bronchial congestion, arthritis, cancers, tumors.

Catalase:

- Enzyme that is the catalyst with SOD in converting hydrogen peroxide into water and oxygen.
- Found in wheat sprouts.
- Potent natural antioxidant.
- May help with fibromyalgia.
- May be helpful in chronic fatigue syndrome.
- Breaks down harmful toxins.

Cauliflower:

- Rich in organic calcium and potassium leading to heart benefits.
- Counters anemia.
- Aids in fever.
- Recommended in cancer prevention.
- Helps to stimulate a stagnant liver.
- Lowers risk of heart disease and stroke.
- Regulates blood pressure.
- Nutritional Facts:
  - Serving Size – 3.5 oz.
  - Calories – 25
  - Fat – 0 g
  - Dietary Fiber – 2 g
  - Sugars – 2g
  - Protein – 2 g

Cayenne pepper:

- Rich source of vitamin A and C.
- Contains very high levels of essential minerals.
- Aids digestion, elimination and assimilation.
- Strong medicine for heart health
- Strong catalyst for all other herbs.
- Powerful stimulant which increases circulation.
- It stops bleeding and regulates blood pressure.
- Studies indicate it kills prostate cancer cells.

Celery:

- Rich source of flavonoid antioxidants which are cancer protective and immune-boosting.
- Good source of vitamin A which helps protect from lung and oral cavity cancers.
- Rich in vitamin C and folic acid and others.
- Excellent source of vitamin K which has established role in limiting neuronal damage in the brain.
- Good source of minerals like potassium which helps control heart rate and blood pressure.

- Essential oils that sooth nervousness, osteoarthritis and gouty-arthritis conditions.
- Have diuretic (removes excess water), stimulant and tonic properties.
- Nutritional Facts:
    - Serving Size – 3.9 oz.
    - Calories – 15
    - Fat – 0 g
    - Dietary Fiber – 2 g
    - Sugars – 2g
    - Protein – 0 g

Celery / (Seed):

- Used to reduce blood pressure.
- Known for its sedative effect.
- May act as an antioxidant.
- A safer diuretic
- Used to help with muscle spasms.
- Helpful for arthritis.
- Has an anti-inflammatory effect.

Cellulose:

- Main ingredient making up plant fiber.
- Vegetable source of fiber.
- Cleans digestive system by bulking waste.
- Sweeps sides of intestines to remove build up.

Chamomile Extract:

- Excellent nerve tonic, sedative and sleep aid.
- Anti-inflammatory.
- Helps with numerous digestive disorders including colitis, and diverticulitis.
- Assists in digestion.
- Antispasmodic used for headaches, fever, muscle cramps and pain.
- Been used to treat rheumatism and arthritis.
- Helps alleviate symptoms of cold, and asthma.

Cheese:

- **Heart smart food**.
- Good amount of calcium which helps control blood pressure.

Cherry:

- Rich in antioxidant properties.
- Very rich in melatonin which helps calm nervous system.
- Regulates heart rate and blood pressure.
- Nutritional Facts:
    - Serving Size – 5.0 oz.
    - Calories – 100
    - Fat – 0g

- Dietary Fiber – 1 g
- Sugars – 16 g
- Protein – 1 g

Chestnut:

- Good source of dietary fiber.
- Rich in vitamin C.
- Rich in folates help to prevent neural tube defects in the fetus.
- Rich source of mono-unsaturated fatty acids. These help prevent coronary artery disease and strokes.
- Gluten-free.
- Nutritional Facts:
  - Serving Size – 10
  - Calories –206
  - Dietary Fiber – 4.3 g
  - Protein – 2.6 g

Chia seeds:

- Good source of omega-3 ALA. Anti-inflammatory helps lower risk of blood pressure, coronary artery disease, strokes, and breast, colon, and prostate cancers.
- Good source of dietary fiber.
- Gluten free.
- Helps benefits individuals with diabetes.
- Good source of niacin which helps reduce LDL-cholesterol levels. It also helps

reduce anxiety and neurosis.

Chili peppers:

- Contain health benefiting compound capsaicin. Has anti-bacterial, anti-carcinogenic, analgesic and anti-diabetic properties.
- Rich in vitamin C.
- Good source of vitamin A.
- Good amount of minerals like potassium and manganese. Potassium helps control heart rate and blood pressure.
- Also good in B-complex vitamins.

Chives:

- Rich in antioxidants that reduces cholesterol and have anti-bacterial, anti-viral, and anti-fungal activities.
- Helps release nitric oxide to decrease blood vessel stiffness.
- Rich in vitamin A which protects from lung and oral cavity cancers.
- Good amount of vitamin C and K to help limiting neuronal damage in the brain.
- Packed with B-complex vitamins.

Chlorella:

- **Is considered a super food.**

- Is called "the world's greatest healthy aging food."
- Chlorella is single-cell, water grown green algae.
- A complete food.
- Has more Vitamin B12 than liver.
- Edible form of water grown algae.
- Helps in cleansing the blood stream.

Cholecalciferol (Vitamin D3):

- **Is considered a Power Nutrient**.
- It is the type of vitamin D that is recommended and should be taken daily.
- Important for calcium and phosphorus absorption, which is necessary for normal growth and development.
- Helps synthesize the enzymes in the mucous membranes that transport calcium.
- Maintains stable nervous system and normal heart action and blood clotting.
- Prevents rickets and osteoporosis.

Choline:

- Choline occurs in a wide variety of foods, including meat, fish, eggs, dairy products, peanuts, broccoli and Brussels sprouts.
- Necessary for nerve function and fat metabolism.
- Protects against poor growth, fatty liver,

and renal damage.

Chromium:

- Chromium is a chemical element found in everyday food like meat, poultry, fish and whole grains.
- Produces energy.
- Regulates blood sugar levels in diabetics.
- Synthesizes cholesterol, fats, and proteins.

Chromium (Chromium Nicotinate):

- Form of chromium.
- Aids in energy metabolism.
- Helps regulate blood sugar in diabetics.
- Reduces effects of heart disease.

Chromium Amino Acid Chelate:

- Amino acid chelate is formed by combining one or more amino acids with the chromium in a chelation reaction.
- Thought by some to be more bio-active than regular chromium hence more readily absorbed by the body.
- Aids in energy metabolism.
- Helps regulate blood sugar in diabetics.
- Reduces effects of heart disease.

Chromium Picolinate:

- **Is a Power Nutrient.**
- It is a combination of chromium and picolinate acid.
- Aids in weight management by promoting the maintenance of lean muscle and the loss of body fat.
- Can help decrease cravings for carbohydrate-rich foods.
- Helps in treatment of metabolic syndrome and type 2 diabetes.
- Helps in treating cardiovascular dysfunction
- Helps treating symptom of clinical depression.
- Chromium picolinate can affect or be affected by the following nutrients:
  - Biotin- adding biotin to chromium can improve the management of blood sugar levels in type 2 diabetics.
  - Vitamin E – can improve insulin function, enhancing the effects of chromium.
  - Manganese – its presence may further enhance the ability of chromium to regulate blood sugar.
- Recommended supplementation 200 mcg per day as a maintenance dosed. 500 to 1,000 mcg per day for weight management, metabolic syndrome, type 2 diabetes and cardiovascular dysfunction.

Cilantro (coriander):

- Rich in antioxidants, essential oils, vitamins, and dietary fiber.
- Vitamin A to protect from lung and oral cavity cancers.
- Rich in vitamin K to protect neuronal damage in the brain.

Cinnamon:

- Source of major antioxidant *catechins.*
- Highest antioxidant strength of all the food sources in nature.
- Essential oils local anesthetic and antiseptic properties, useful in dental and gum treatment.
- Anti-clotting action, prevent platelet clogging inside blood vessels.
- Stimulates peripheral circulation.
- Relieves spasms.
- Helps lower fevers.
- Known to lower blood pressure.
- Helps to control bleeding.
- Helps control infections.
- Improves digestion.
- Treatment for diarrhea.
- Helps check candida.
- Relieves pain of arthritis and rheumatism.

- Works to relieve cold and flu symptoms.
- Useful as a flavoring.

Citrulline:

- **Is an amino acid and is considered a Power Nutrient**.
- Has performance-enhancing effects and to reduce muscle fatigue.
- Involved in maintaining nitrogen balance in the body.
- Involved in supporting metabolism.
- Its major benefit is being converted into arginine, the powerful amino acid that produces nitric oxide.
- Recommended supplementation of 500 to 2,000 mg daily for optimal cardiovascular benefits.

Citrus:

- Major source of antioxidants *flavonoids* and *Vitamin C*.

Citrus Bioflavonoids:

- **Is an antioxidant which is considered a Power Nutrient.**
- Major antioxidant found in citrus fruits.
- Critical to the proper absorption and use of Vitamin C.

- Keeps collagen (intercellular cement) healthy.
- Increases the strength and permeability of capillaries.
- Forms protective barrier against infections.
- Lowers cholesterol levels.
- Vitamin P complex.
- Maintains blood vessel walls.
- Used as a reducing agent.

Citrus Pectin:

- Useful for balancing acid / alkaline levels.
- Slows the absorption of food. Allowing the removal of unwanted metals and toxins.
- Lowers cholesterol and reduces occurrence of heart disease.

Clove Oil:

- Useful as an antiseptic, anti-bacterial and anti-viral agent.
- May be helpful with premature ejaculation.
- Useful in lowering fever.
- Helpful in preventing the formation of dry sockets after tooth extraction.

Clover Extract:

- Red clover is a species native to Europe, Western Asia and northwest Africa.
- Used as a blood purifier.
- Has antispasmodic properties.
- Makes a good sedative to relax muscle cramping and nervous exhaustion.
- Relieves irritation and inflammation of the urinary tract.
- Used for menopausal problems.
- Wonderful for scrofulous and skin diseases.
- Great antidote for cancer.
- Helps bronchitis, leprosy, syphilis, rickets, indolent ulcers.

Cloves:

- Relieves pain.
- Controls nausea and vomiting.
- Improves digestion.
- Works as an antiseptic.
- Useful as a kidney tonic.
- Helps control parasites.
- Helpful with hiccups.
- Treatment for impotence.
- Aids those with hypoglycemia.

Coconut:

- Has important saturated fatty acid, lauric acid which benefits cholesterol levels.

- Coconut water has enzymes which aid in digestion and metabolism.
- Excellent source of a number of needed minerals.
- Good source of B-complex vitamins.
- Nutritional Facts:
  - Serving Size – 1 C
  - Calories –283
  - Dietary Fiber – 7.2 g
  - Protein – 2.6 g

Coenzyme Q10 (CoQ10)

- **Is considered a Power Nutrient.**
- The second most important nutrient in the cardiovascular system after nitric oxide.
- 75% of cardiovascular patients are deficient in CoQ10.
- 39% of patients with high blood pressure are deficient in CoQ10.
- Statin drugs deplete the body of CoQ10.
- Involved in production of energy from fat.
- Functions as an antioxidant, especially in the cardiovascular system.
- CoQ10 confers benefits related to obesity, metabolic syndrome, diabetes, cardiovascular dysfunction, immune health, gum disease, and Parkinson's Disease.
- Recommended supplementation: for optimal health - 100 to 200 mg per day. Those with obesity, diabetes or

cardiovascular dysfunction – 400 mg per day. Those with Parkinson's disease – 1,200 mg per day.

Cohosh Extract:

- Induces labor.
- Good for morning sickness.
- Anti-inflammatory.
- Antispasmodic.
- Good for anorexia.
- Helps reduce anxiety.
- Relieves coughing.
- Delays degeneration of the retina.
- Relieves fibrositis, headaches, hot flashes, hysteria, myalgia, PMS, arthritis, & uterine cramps.
- Lowers blood pressure and cholesterol.

Collard greens:

- Good source of vitamin A, C, K and B-complex.
- Rich in phyto-nutrients that benefit prostate, breast, cervical, colon, and ovarian cancers.
- Excellent source of folates which help prevent neural tube defects in babies.
- Protects against flu-like viral infections.

Cooking Oil:

Below (next page) is a table with in-depth analysis of some commonly used dietary fats and oils:

Item	SFA %	MUFA %	PUFA% ω-6 ω-3		ω-6 to ω-3 ratio	Remarks
Canola	8	61	21	10	2:1	Recommended
Flax seed oil	9	18	16	57	1:3.5	Recommended
Safflower	10	13	77	0	77:0	Somewhat recommended
Sunflower	11	20	69	0	69:0	Somewhat recommended
Olive	14	77	8	1	8:1	Highly recommended
Soybean	15	25	53	7	8:1	Recommended
Sesame	15	42	43	0	43:0	Recommended
Peanut	18	49	33	0	33:0	Recommended
Salmon fat	24	34	0	42	0:42	Somewhat recommended
Cotton seed	27	19	54	0	54:0	Somewhat recommended

Chicken fat	32	47	21	0	21:0	Somewhat recommended
Palm oil	40	48	11	1	11:1	Somewhat recommended
Pork fat	41	48	11	0	11:0	Not recommended
Beef tallow	47	53	0	0	0:0	Not recommended
Cocoa butter	64	31	0	0	0:0	Not recommended
Butter	69	31	0	0	0:0	Not recommended
Cheese	70	30	0	0	0:0	Not recommended
Hydrogenated vegetable oil	76	19	0	0	0:0	Not recommended
Coconut oil	92	6	1.6	0.4	4:0	Not recommended

SFA=Saturated fatty acids

MUFA=Mono-unsaturated fatty acids

PUFA=Poly-unsaturated fatty acids

ω-3=Omega 3 fatty acids

ω-6=Omega 6 fatty acids

Copper:

- Trace mineral essential to bone formation and maintenance of healthy nerves.
- Facilitates iron absorption, hemoglobin, and red blood cells.
- Helps body to oxidize Vitamin C.
- Works with zinc and Vitamin C to form elastin.
- Aids in the production of RNA.
- Scientific literature supports the theory that copper deficiency is related to aortic aneurysm and atherosclerotic vascular disease or heart disease.

Coriander seeds:

- Rich in dietary fiber.
- Excellent source of minerals like iron and

potassium.
- Contain vitamin C.
- Good amount of vital B-complex.
- Essential oils are responsible for digestive, carinative and anti-flatulent properties.

Cordyceps Extract, Dried:

- Cordyceps is a genus of sac fungi.
- Ancient Chinese tonic herb (Cordyceps Sinensis) traditionally used to increase strength, endurance, male potency and female vitality.
- Benefits the circulatory, immune, respiratory, and glandular systems.

Corn:

- **Heart smart food**.
- Good source of folic acid.
- Protects arteries.
- Gluten free.
- High-quality phyto-nutrition.
- Good source of flavonoid antioxidant.
- Nutritional Facts:
    - Serving Size – 3.2oz.
    - Calories – 90
    - Fat – 2.5 g
    - Dietary Fiber – 2 g
    - Sugars – 5 g
    - Protein – 4 g

Corn Bran Fiber:

- Source of fiber from corn which is higher than wheat in nutrients, especially zinc.
- Shown to lower cholesterol levels.

Corn Gluten, Hydrolyzed:

- Process of turning corn gluten into a more "watery" substance or simpler compound.
- A nutrient supplement.
- Rich in protein.

Corn Silk Extract, Dried (Silks):

- Diuretic.
- Helps all urinary tract complaints.

Corn Starch:

- Used because of its absorbency.
- Helps soothe irritated membranes such as the colon.
- Useful as a safe diuretic.
- Useful as a thickening agent.
- Sometimes used to line containers to keep products from sticking to the sides.

Cranberry and Extract:

- Good source of vitamin A and C.
- Keeps bacteria such as e-coli from sticking

to the bladder.
- Beneficial for urinary tract infections and other infections like E-coli.
- Helpful in the recovery from stroke.
- Could be helpful in significantly reducing the loss of brain cells.
- Limits LDL build up.
- Helpful with cardiovascular disease.
- May prevent and even improve skin conditions in people with urinary wall disease.
- Has: anti-inflammatory, anti-cancer, and chemotherapeutic properties as a result of reservatrol, an antioxidant.
- Helpful in reducing infections that may be caused by users of catheters.
- **Caution should be used when using cranberry juice while using the drug Warfarin.

Cucumber:

- Have a mild diuretic property to help with blood pressure and weight management.
- High amount of vitamin K helps with bone mass and treatment of Alzheimer's.
- Nutritional Facts:
    - Serving Size – 3.5 oz.
    - Calories – 10
    - Fat – 0 g
    - Dietary Fiber – 1 g
    - Sugars – 1g
    - Protein – 1 g

Cumin seeds:

- Active principles in cumin may augment the motility of the gastro-intestinal tract as well as aids the digest power.
- Excellent source of minerals like iron, potassium and selenium.
- Rich source of many flavonoid antioxidants.

Cupric Oxide (Copper):

- Trace mineral essential to bone formation and maintenance of healthy nerves.
- Facilitates iron absorption, hemoglobin, and red blood cells.
- Helps body to oxidize Vitamin C.
- Works with zinc and Vitamin C to form elastin.
- Aids in the production of RNA.
- Scientific literature supports the theory that copper deficiency is related to aortic aneurysm and atherosclerotic vascular disease or heart disease.
- Current information does not indicate that any of the various forms of copper such as amino acid chelate, Gluconate, etc., have a better result than the other.

Curcuma Longa:

- A member of the ginger family.
- Also known as Turmeric.

- Adds flavor.
- Improves digestion.
- Stimulates circulation.
- Relaxes spasms.
- Alleviates pain.
- Aids in indigestion, low blood pressure, colic, morning sickness, flu.
- Helpful with neurogenous diseases such as multiple sclerosis.
- Used to treat flatulence, jaundice, menstrual problems, and hemorrhage.
- Inhibits production of inflammation related enzymes which are found in cancers, especially bowel and colon and certain inflammatory diseases
- Acts as an antioxidant.
- Prevents free radical damage.
- Improves rheumatoid arthritis.
- Improves respiratory disorders.

Cyanocobalamin (Vitamin B12) :
- Important in cell formation and longevity.
- Prevents anemia.
- Counters nerve damage and maintains fertility.
- Aids greatly in digestion and absorption process.
- Found to increase energy.
- Helps to restore mental abilities dealing with memory loss and mental clarity.

- Helps to deal with stress.
- Calms irritability.
- Helps prevent diabetic complications.

Cysteine:

- **Is an amino acid and is considered a Power Nutrient**.
- Essential for infants, the elderly, and individuals with certain metabolic diseases or who suffer from malabsorption syndromes.
- Powerful detoxifying agent that helps the body recover from the toxins created by alcohol consumption and tobacco use.
- Strengthens the immune system.
- Acts as the body's chief antioxidant
- Directs the functions of other antioxidants and helps molecules like Vitamins E and C be more effective at preventing oxidative damage to cells.
- Recommended supplementation of 250 to 1,500 mg daily for antioxidant support.

D-Alpha Tocopherol (Vitamin E):

- **Is an antioxidant which is considered a Power Nutrient.**
- Is a powerful fat soluble antioxidant.
- Key to cellular respiration.
- Prevents cell damage and repairs tissue while reducing scarring.

- Critical to the normal clotting of the blood
.
- Strengthens capillary walls and produces red blood cells.
- Seems to have a dramatic effect on the reproductive system of both males and females.
- Can be a diuretic to the system.
- Seems to reduce coronary heart disease.
- This form of Vitamin E is linked to inflammation reduction.
- Seems to diminish arthritic pain.
- Used in conjunction with Vitamin C in the treatment of cataracts.
- Helps control epileptic seizures.
- Helps cause the disappearance of granuloma annulare, a skin disease.
- Improves glucose tolerance and insulin sensitivity, especially in diabetics.
- Useful in stabilizing patients with chronic skin ulcers.
- Useful in reducing heavy blood flow in females.
- Optimal level of intake of this form of Vitamin E is 400 IU. The RDA is only 30 IU.
- **You would need to eat 33 heads of spinach, 27 lbs. of butter, 80 avocados, or 5 lbs. of wheat germ every day to obtain 400 IU of Vitamin E.

D-Calcium Pantothenate:

- Also called pantothenate or vitaminB_5.
- Small quantities found in most foods, especially meat.
- Wonderful aid in healing wounds.
- Critical to cell metabolism.
- Releases energy from carbohydrates, fats, and proteins.
- Reduces toxic effects of antibiotics.
- Fights infection.
- Builds antibodies.
- Helps prevent fatigue.
- Reverses toxic effects of many antibodies.
- Good for hypoglycemia, ulcers, and blood and skin disorders.

Dandelion (Leaf):

- An effective diuretic.
- Rich in potassium.
- Helps alleviate fluid retention, especially with heart problems.
- Good for other urinary disorders.
- Effective liver and digestive tonic.
- Helps with cirrhosis of the liver.
- Strengthens kidney, spleen and pancreas.
- Helps hepatitis and jaundice.
- May reduce aging spots.
- Fights against breast cancer.
- Increases bile production.

- Cleanses blood and liver.

Dandelion Root:

- A blood purifier and diuretic.
- Enhances liver function by balancing digestive enzymes.
- Helps with hepatitis, hypoglycemia.
- Lowers cholesterol, blood pressure.
- High in calcium and iron.

Dark chocolate:

- **Heart smart food**.
- **Brain booster**.
- A source of major antioxidant *epicatechin*.
- Contains phenols.
- You need at least 80% cacao in order to receive all the health benefits.
- Increase immune system.
- Reduce colon cancer risk.
- Protection against heart and cardiovascular disease.
- Regulation of blood sugar.
- Slows aging.
- DNA repair and protection.
- Alleviation of high blood pressure
- Promotion of eye health.
- Osteoporosis protection.
- Reduced frequency of migraine headache.

- Alleviation of PMS.
- Alleviation of common cold.

Dates:

- Rich in dietary fiber.
- Moderate source of vitamin A.
- Good source of B-complex and vitamin K.
- Helps prevent colon, lung, prostate, breast, endometrial and pancreatic cancers.
- Offers protection against stroke and heart diseases.
- Helps protects against some age related eye conditions.

De-Fatted Peanut Flour, Partially:

- Derived from removing a percentage of the oil from the peanut, drying it and then turning it into meal or flour.
- Process extends the shelf life.
- Maintains rich peanut butter flavor while providing a well-balanced protein.

DHA (Docosahexaenoic Acid):

- Part of Omega-3 which is considered a Power Nutrient.
- Omega 3 long chain polyunsaturated fat.

- Essential for growth and functional development in infants brains and maintenance of the adult brain.
- Helps with memory loss and vision problems.
- Shown to help with inflammation in Crohn's disease and rheumatoid arthritis.
- May also help with kidney diseases and chronic obstructive pulmonary disease.
- Helps maintain triglyceride levels.
- DHA has a positive effect on diseases such as hypertension, arthritis, atherosclerosis, depression, adult-onset diabetes mellitus, myocardial infarction, thrombosis, and some cancers.

Dill:

- Rich in vital vitamins like A and C which help protect from lung and oral cavity cancers.
- Good source of minerals which regulate digestion, control heart rate and blood pressure.

DL-Alpha...Tocopheryl Acetate (Vitamin E):

- **Is a powerful antioxidant which is considered a Power Nutrient**
- Synthetic form of Vitamin E.

- Key to cellular respiration.
- Prevents cell damage and repairs tissue while reducing scarring.
- Critical to the normal clotting of the blood.
- Strengthens capillary walls and produces red blood cells.
- Seems to have a dramatic effect on the reproductive system of both males and females.
- Can be a diuretic to the system.

DL-Methionine:

- **Is an amino acid and is considered a Power Nutrient**.
- Amino acid that aids in breakdown of fats, preventing buildup especially in liver and arteries.
- Produces brain food (choline).
- Helps digestive process, prevents toxemia in pregnancy.
- Detoxicant for chemicals and other environmental pollutants.

Docosahexaenoic Acid (DHA):

- Omega 3 long chain polyunsaturated fat.
- Essential for growth and functional development in infants brains and maintenance of the adult brain.

- Helps with memory loss and vision problems.
- Shown to help with inflammation in Crohn's disease and rheumatoid arthritis.
- May also help with kidney diseases and chronic obstructive pulmonary disease.
- Helps maintain triglyceride levels.
- DHA has a positive effect on diseases such as hypertension, arthritis, atherosclerosis, depression, adult-onset diabetes mellitus, myocardial infarction, thrombosis, and some cancers.

Echinacea:

- Beneficial herb for acute infection.
- Aids the digestive system.
- Helps the female reproductive system.
- Beneficial to the excretory system.
- Improves immune system.
- Great to take when you feel a cold coming on.

Egg Albumin Solids Powder:

- A group of simple proteins used as an emulsifier in foods and cosmetics.

Eggs:

- Excellent source of protein.
- Provides Vitamins A, B1, B2, B6, Bl2, D and E.

- Good source of minerals: Iron, Zinc,
- Calcium, Iodine, and Selenium.
- Contains polyunsaturated fat which helps to lower cholesterol.

Eicosapentaenoic Acid (EPA):

- Essential Omega-3 fatty acid found in fish oil.
- Helps with cardiovascular disease, i.e.
- Chrons disease, cancer, and many others.

Eleuthero Extract, Dried (Siberian Ginseng) (Root):

- Small woody shrub native to northeastern Asia.
- Enhances endurance.
- Increases/decreases cell division.
- Protects against toxicity, especially radiation.
- Stimulates male sex glands.
- Chinese consider this the best treatment for insomnia.
- Extensively used for bronchitis and chronic lung ailments.
- Helps in treatment of heart disease and high blood pressure.
- Aids in the reduction of cholesterol levels.
- Useful in treating arthritis, low blood oxygen, impotence, and stress.

English Lavender (Flower):

- Relaxes spasms and has antidepressant abilities.
- Medically used for depression, anxiety, exhaustion, irritability, and insomnia.

Ergocalciferol (Vitamin D2):

- Used as a food product enhancer.
- Speeds up body's production of calcium.
- Lack of can lead to rickets and bone deterioration.
- Aids in absorption of calcium and the assimilation of phosphorous which is required for bone formation.
- Helps synthesize the enzymes in the mucous membranes that transport calcium.
- Maintains s stable nervous system and normal heart action and blood clotting.

Fennel:

- Rich source of dietary fiber.
- Has anti-fungal and anti-bacterial properties.
- Has vitamins and minerals that are essential for optimum health.
- Strong appetite suppressant, stimulates

energy production.
- Antacid, antispasmodic, and expectorant.
- Increases secretion of mother's milk.
- A safer diuretic.

Fenugreek:

- Fenugreek is an annual plant that is cultivated worldwide.
- Useful for all mucous conditions and lung congestion.
- Helps with ulcers, inflamed stomach, and intestinal conditions.
- Used also in the treatment of diabetes and gout.
- Aids in eliminating boils and carbuncles.

Filbert:

- (see Hazelnuts)

Fish Oils (Marine Lipid Complex) (Eicosapentanoic Acid (EPA)) & (Docosahexaenoic Acid (DHA)):

- Helps to lubricate joints.
- Provides healthy brain cell tissue.
- Found to help children with attention deficit disorder.
- Promotes mental clarity and "good vibrations" (mood).
- Great for the heart (tends to lower

cholesterol and promote a healthy inflammation response as measured for C-reactive protein levels).
- See "Omega-3 Fatty Acids".
- See "Eicosapentaenoic Acid (EPA)".
- See "Docosahexaenoic Acid (DHA)".

Flax seed:

- Rich in monounsaturated fatty acids which help prevent coronary artery disease and strokes.
- Good source of omega-3 ALA. This then converts in the body to also form EPA. Not as potent as from cold water fish and does not provide the DHA.
- Contains *lignans*, which helps prevent cancer.
- Excellent source of vitamin E.
- Good source of B-complex vitamins.
- Nutritional Facts:
  - Serving Size – 1 T
  - Calories –55
  - Dietary Fiber – 2.8 g
  - Protein – 1.9 g

Folate (Folic Acid) (Vitamin B$_9$):

- Is coenzyme in DNA process of cell division and replication.
- Essential to embryonic and fetal

development and prevention of mental retardation.
- Is a carbon carrier, brain food and increases energy.

Fructooligosaccharides (FOS):

- Sugars that occur naturally in plants. Extracted from bananas, barley, chicory root, etc.
- Commercially used in prepared syrups.
- Not digestible in the stomach so may travel unabsorbed to the intestine.
- Promotes growth of friendly bacteria in the intestines.
- Decreases chances of yeast infection.
- Has been a popular dietary supplement in Japan for a number of years.

Fructose:

- Fructose is fruit sugar.
- Pure, dry fructose is a very sweet, white, odorless, crystalline solid and is the most water-soluble of all sugars.
- Because it does not cause blood sugar to rise much it was once thought that it was a good substitute for sucrose (table sugar). However, studies have caused nutritional experts to change their minds.

- A small amount of fructose, such as the amount found in most vegetables and fruits, is not a bad thing. However, consuming too much fructose at once seems to overwhelm the body's capacity to process it.
- The diets of our ancestors contained only very small amounts of fructose.
- It causes high blood triglycerides which are a risk factor for heart disease.
- It ends up circumventing the normal appetite signaling system, so you can eat too much.
- Studies are also showing it may lead to diabetes.

Fumaric Acid:

- Is found in fumitory in bolete mushrooms.
- Used as a raw material for food additives.
- Used to treat psoriasis.

Garcinia Cambogia:

- Is a small, pumpkin shaped fruit, sometimes called tamarind.
- It is native to Indonesia, it is also grown in India, Southeast Asia, and West and Central Africa.
- Decreases appetite thus helping weight loss.

- Stops synthesis of fat.
- Balances sugar metabolism in diabetes.

Garlic:

- **Heart smart food**.
- Major medicinal herb used for countless proposes.
- Good for all diseases and infections.
- Is a stimulant and powerful antibiotic, antiviral, antifungal and parasiticide.
- Excellent for all heart disorders, especially blood pressure problems.
- Lowers cholesterol.
- Thins blood.
- Good for digestion, asthma.
- Used for colds and flu.
- Used for bronchitis.
- Helpful in treating cholera, dysentery, and typhoid.
- Has compound *allicin* that have anti-bacterial, anti-viral, and anti-fungal activities.
- Supports immune system.

German Chamomile (Flower):

- Grown in the U.S.
- Excellent nerve tonic, sedative and sleep aid.
- Antispasmodic used for headaches, fever,

muscle cramps and pain.
- Been used to treat rheumatism and arthritis.
- Helps alleviate symptoms of cold, and asthma.

Ginger:

- Contains health benefiting essential oils that are anti-inflammatory, analgesic, nerve soothing, anti-bacterial. Reduces motion sickness and relieve migraine headache.
- Chemicals effective against *E.coli* induced diarrhea.
- Good amount of minerals like potassium that helps control heart rate and blood pressure.

Ginger Extract:

- An excellent stimulant which increases metabolism and circulation.
- Effective for colds and flu.
- Breaks up obstructions and promotes sweating.
- Stops bleeding, relieves constipation, good for menstrual cramps.
- Externally used for treating pain and inflammation in joints.

Gingko Biloba Extract (Leaves):

- Herb approved by the German Commission for use in vertigo, tinnitus, intermittent claudication, and dementia.
- Useful in improving memory loss.
- Has neuro protective characteristics.
- Useful antioxidant.

Ginseng Extract, Dried Oriental:

- King of tonics.
- Stimulates entire body energy.
- Cardiovascular regulator and stimulant.

Ginseng Extract, Dried Panax (Root):

- Increases T cell and killer cell activity.
- Increases general sense of well-being.
- Increases mental & physical activity.
- Enhances immune functions.
- May help with blood glucose levels in type 2 diabetes.

Ginseng, Panax (Root):

- Asian Ginseng.
- Studies indicate ginseng is helpful with erectile dysfunction.
- May be helpful with epilepsy.

Glucohydrolase, 4D:

- Originates from barley
- Is an enzyme.
- Shows inhibition of cancer cells in animal studies.

Glucomannan:

- Is a water-soluble dietary fiber.
- Comes from the roots of the konjac plant.
- Picks up and removes fat from colon wall.
- Expands to 60 times its weight which helps curb appetite.
- Normalizes blood sugar and reduces allergic reactions.

Glucosamine Sulfate:

- **Glucosamine is considered a Power Nutrient.**
- Scientific research indicates glucosamine helps with arthritic pain.
- There are no food sources of glucosamine.
- Our body's natural production of glucosamine slows with age.
- Treatment of osteoarthritis.
- Treatment of osteoporosis.
- Injury prevention and exercise performance enhancement.
- Recommended supplementation: 1,500 mg per day. Obese individuals may

require more glucosamine; 20 mg per kilogram of body weight.

Glucose:

- A form of sugar from plants. It is one of three dietary sugars, along with fructose and galactose.
- Glucose is the form of energy the body is designed to run on. Every cell in your body, every bacterium – and in fact, every living thing on Earth – uses glucose for energy.
- Every cell in your body, including your brain, utilizes glucose. Therefore, much of it is "burned up" immediately after you consume it. By contrast, fructose is turned into free fatty acids (FFA), LDL (the damaging form of cholesterol), and triglycerides, which get stored as fat.

Glucosinolates (from Broccoli Sprout Extract):

- Found in cruciferous vegetables.
- Appear to protect against cancer of the lungs and alimentary tract.

Glutamic Acid:

- **Is an amino acid and is considered a Power Nutrient.**

- Primary brain food.
- Increases the firing of neurons in the nervous system.
- Metabolizes sugars and fats.
- Corrects personality disorders.

Glycine:

- **Is an amino acid and is considered a Power Nutrient**.
- Helps trigger the release of oxygen.
- Can produce energy.
- Necessary ingredient for a healthy prostate.
- Necessary ingredient for repairing damaged tissues.

Goldenseal:

- Is a perennial herb in the buttercup family.
- Used as an herbal antibiotic, antibacterial, antiseptic agent.
- Destroys yeast and bacteria in the gastrointestinal tract and clears the flora.
- Its detoxifying agent extends to the circulatory system.
- Sedates and regulates the liver and spleen.
- Helps with sugar metabolism.
- Helps with fat metabolism.
- Purifies mucous membranes.

Gotu Kola:

- Is another name for centella, a small annual plant family native to India and other parts of Asia.
- Stimulates central nervous system.
- Good for brain, memory.
- Decreases fatigue and depression.
- Increases sex drive.
- Has diuretic properties and neutralizes blood acids.

Grapes:

- **Brain booster**.
- Rich in antioxidant resveratrol.
- Helps protect against colon and prostate cancer and heart disease.
- Good source vitamin A, C, K and B-complex.
- **Nutritional Facts:**
  - Serving Size – 4.5 oz.
  - Calories – 90
  - Fat – 0g
  - Dietary Fiber – 1g
  - Sugars – 20g
  - Protein – 0g

Grape Skin Extract:

- **Brain booster.**

- May help lessen the damage to the brain during and after strokes.
- Contains *reservatrol* which is known to be helpful with atherosclerosis.
- Helpful in protecting against breast cancer.
- May be helpful in reducing skin cancer.
- Studies indicate it may be useful in fighting against lung inflammation.

Grapefruit:

- **Heart smart food**.
- Bioflavonoid moves and regulates the spleen / pancreas digestive energy.
- Very good source of vitamin A and C.
- Helps resolve mucous conditions of the lungs.
- Works to detoxify.
- Helps alleviate intestinal gas, pain and swelling.
- Useful in strengthening gums.
- Strengthen arteries and aids circulation.
- **Nutritional Facts:**
  - Serving Size – 5.5 oz.
  - Calories –60
  - Fat – 0g
  - Dietary Fiber – 2g
  - Sugars – 11g
  - Protein – 1g

Green beans:

- Rich source of dietary fiber.
- Excellent levels of vitamin A.
- Good source of important folates.
- Good source of Vitamins B_6 and C.
- Nutritional Facts:
    - Serving Size – 3.0 oz.
    - Calories – 20
    - Fat – 0 g
    - Dietary Fiber – 3 g
    - Sugars – 2g
    - Protein – 1 g

Green leafy vegetables:

- Source of major antioxidant *carotenoids*.
- **Brain booster**.
- Lettuces which are rich in vitamins A, C and K. Eating regularly will improve your eyesight, bone health and skin elasticity while helping your blood to clot normally.
- Cruciferous greens like Kale, mustard greens cabbage etc. are high in nutrients and contain glucosinolates, which inhibit the growth of certain cancers. Various minerals enhance heart health and brain function.
- Spinach and Swiss Chard are rich in iron, which carries oxygen to the blood.
- Edible green leaves like dandelion, red clover and watercress promote a healthy liver, keep skin cells healthy and have anti-inflammatory properties.

Green Onion:

- Used for flavoring.
- Boosts friendly bacteria and immune system.
- Contains sulfides known to lower blood pressure and blood lipids.
- Onions in general have an anti-tumor effect.
- Study indicated decrease in stomach cancer when large quantities of onions were consumed.
- Uncontrolled studies showed onions can lower sugar levels in diabetes.
- Other studies show that onions may help with asthma, eczema, coughs and infections.
- Nutritional Facts:
    - Serving Size – 0.9 oz.
    - Calories – 10
    - Fat – 0 g
    - Dietary Fiber – 1 g
    - Sugars – 1g
    - Protein – 0 g

Green Tea:

- **Green tea is considered a Power Nutrient.**
- **Heart smart food.**

- **Brain booster**.
- Source of major antioxidant *catechins*.
- The primary antioxidant in green tea (EGCG) is 100 times more potent than vitamins C and E.
- One cup of green tea (delivering 10-40 mg of antioxidant polyphenols) has antioxidant effects greater than a serving of broccoli, spinach or carrots.
- Green tea has the highest polyphenol content with less than a third the caffeine of black tea.
- Also known as Camellia Sinensis.
- Increases energy thus helping to burn more calories and fat, thus helping obesity and weight management.
- Immune support and general vitality.
- Effective as an antiviral and antioxidant.
- Helps shield against tumors of the liver, lung, skin, and digestive tract.
- Stabilizes blood lipids and lowers cholesterol.
- Extremely useful in treatment of cardiovascular dysfunction.
- Helps with metabolic syndrome and type 2 diabetes treatment.
- Effective in cancer prevention.
- Helps HIV.
- Helps with periodontal disease.
- Protects the body from cancer.
- May help in regulating blood sugar levels

thus could be useful for diabetics.

- Recommended supplementation: for general health promotion, two to three cups of green tea per day (a total of 2240 to 320 mg of polyphenols)

Guar Gum:

- Ground endosperm from guar beans.
- Botanical root which curbs appetite thus helpful with weight loss.
- Reduces cholesterol and triglyceride levels.
- Binds toxic substances and carries them out of the body.

Guarana (Seed):

- Guarana is a climbing plant native to the Amazon basin.
- Natural source of caffeine processed differently from commercial caffeine. Approximately 4% naturally occurring caffeine.
- It enters and leaves the body more slowly, leaves no residues in liver and is not isolated or processed like caffeine.
- Stimulates energy levels.
- Guaranine is the active ingredient in guarana that is similar to caffeine.
- Used for arthritis.

- Useful in controlling diarrhea.

Gum Arabic:

- Gum from the Acacia tree.
- Dissolves rapidly in water.
- Retards sugar from crystallizing.
- Used as a thickener for candy and gum.
- Prevents chemical breakdown in foods.
- Gives form and shape to tablets.
- Used for dysentery and diarrhea.

Gymnena Sylvestre Extract, Dried (Leaves):

- An herb native to the tropical forests of southern and central India.
- Helpful in diabetes by controlling insulin.
- May be helpful in stomach problems
- Can be helpful when used for constipation.

Hawthorn Berry:

- Dilates coronary vessels.
- Aids angina.
- Helps speed recovery from heart attack.
- Lowers cholesterol.
- Regenerates heart muscle walls.
- Increases calcium absorption, thus is excellent for broken bones, tissue, teeth, nails, and hair.

- Used for Alzheimer's disease.
- Opens capillaries so more oxygen and nutrients get to the brain.
- Helps with attention deficit disorder.
- Laboratory studies show that it helps with diabetic retinopathy and other eye disorders.
- Lab studies show strong indications of helpfulness with leukemia, throat cancer, and lupus.
- **Caution** Always use competent medical care when dealing with serious heart and cancer situations, and when dealing with pregnant and nursing mothers.

Hazelnut:

- Very high in energy.
- Rich in dietary fiber.
- Rich in folate.
- Excellent source of vitamin E.
- Gluten free.
- Helps prevent some cancers, coronary artery disease and strokes.
- Nutritional Facts:
    - Serving Size – 1 oz.
    - Calories –178
    - Dietary Fiber – 2.7 g
    - Protein – 4.2 g

Hesperidin:

- Hesperidin is a flavanone glycoside found abundantly in citrus fruits.
- Critical to proper absorption and use of Vitamin C.
- Keeps collagen (intercellular cement) healthy.
- Increases strength and permeability of capillaries.
- Forms protective barrier against infections.
- Lowers cholesterol.

Hibiscus Flower Powder:

- Anti-inflammatory.
- Useful in treating fevers.
- Fights heart disease.
- May lower bad cholesterol.
- Helps lower blood pressure.

Hippohae Rhamnoides:

- Hippophae rhamnoides, common sea-buckthorn, is a species of flowering plant in the family Elaeagnaceae, native to fixed dunes and sea cliffs in Europe and Asia
- Rich in Rose Hips Acerola, and Vitamins A, B12, C & E.
- The berries carry a high content of essential fatty acids.
- The combination of Vitamin B12 and

Vitamin C work perfectly to enhance metabolic functioning.
- Known and used extensively to maintain healthy skin.
- Protects the healthy mucus of the stomach and acts as an anti-inflammatory.
- Promotes tissue regeneration.
- Helps with stomach ulcers.
- Reduces cholesterol.
- Shows anti-cancer activity.
- Inhibits platelet aggregation.

Honey:
- Known as a complete food.
- Honey is high in protein, carbohydrates, vitamins, and some minerals.
- Promotes energy and healing.

Hops Extract, Dried:
- Known as a potent sedative.
- Relieves pain.
- Relaxes spasms.
- Regulates hormones.
- Relieves insomnia.
- Works on irritable bowel syndrome.
- **Caution** May cause depression.

Horsetail Herb:

- Horsetail (Equisetum arvense) is an herbal remedy dating back to ancient Roman and Greek medicine.
- Increases calcium absorption.
- Strengthens hair, nails, and bones.
- Is diuretic and hemostatic (stops bleeding).
- Used to treat kidney stones.

Horseradish:

- Contains many volatile compounds found to have antioxidant as well as detoxification functions.
- Facilitates digestions.
- Good amount of vitamin C.
- Has vital minerals like potassium.

Hydrangea (Root):

- Used primarily as a pain killer for both muscles and bones.
- Strengthens and increases circulation in joints and muscles.

Inositol:

- Inositol is a substance that is naturally present in human cells and in certain foods. It is also available in supplement form (which is where I find the best

available)
- It is very beneficial for cellular nutrition.
- Water soluble.
- Combines with choline to form lecithin.
- Found more in the body than any other vitamin except niacin.
- Abundant in the heart muscle and brain.
- The "brain nourisher."
- Helps Vitamin E utilization.
- Prevents hardening of the arteries.
- Lowers and controls cholesterol levels.
- Synergistic with Vitamin E in treating nerve damage.
- Helps cerebral palsy.
- Aids in muscular dystrophy.
- Helps to metabolize fat.
- Important in hair growth.   Prevents baldness.

Inulin:

- A polysaccharide derived from the Jerusalem artichoke and Dahlia Tuber.
- Formed by linking 30 fructose monomer units together in a long chain.
- Natural fiber that helps to moderate blood sugar levels in the body.
- May reduce sugar cravings.
- Not absorbed by digestive tract and therefore does not contribute any calories while improving energy levels.

Iodine (As Potassium Iodide):

- Important to physical and mental development.
- Metabolizes excess fat, creates energy and increases metabolic rate.
- Regulates thyroid.

Iron:

- Combines with protein and copper to form hemoglobin which transports oxygen to blood from lungs to tissues (muscles).
- Increases resistance to stress and disease.
- Metabolizes protein, helps in energy production.
- Also used as additive for coloring.

Isolated Soy Protein:

- Provides most of the essential amino acids.
- No cholesterol.
- Low in fat.
- Has isoflavones which are antioxidants and may help with menopause symptoms
- May reduce the risk of hormone dependent cancers.
- Provides genistein and daidzein.
- Promotes healthy blood serum

cholesterol.

Jalapeno peppers:

- Contains compounds like capsaicin which is found to have anti-bacterial, anti-carcinogenic, analgesic, and anti-diabetic properties.
- Also found to reduce LDL-cholesterol levels.
- Rich source of vitamin C.
- Contain vitamin A and other valuable antioxidants.
- Contain good amount of vitamin E and K.

Jicama:

- Great source of dietary fiber.
- Rich in vitamin C.

Jujube Extract:

- Chinese Herb.
- Scientific name, Ziziphus Spinosa.
- Contains flavonoids and saponins and glycosides.
- Seeds have known sedative activity.
- Signs of protective qualities against radioactive damage.
- Shown to protect myocardial (heart) cells from oxygen and glucose deprivation .
- Used to control allergic reactions.
- Relieves coughing.

- Alleviates nervous breakdown.
- Can calm irritability.

Kale:

- Rich in vitamin A, C and K.
- Good amounts of B-complex.
- Helps protect against prostate and colon cancers.
- Helps prevent retinal detachment and macular degeneration.

Kelp:

- Type of seaweed which is rich source of minerals, vitamins, and trace elements, especially iron.
- Used as flavoring and salt substitute.
- Good for thyroid and obesity.
- Beneficial to sensory nerves and membranes that surround the brain and spinal cord.

Kiwi:

- Excellent source of vitamin A, C, E, and K.
- Helps prevent some cancers.
- Excellent source of omega-3.
- Rich in heart-healthy potassium.
- **Nutritional Facts:**
  - Serving Size – 5.3 oz.
  - Calories – 90
  - Fat – 1g

- Dietary Fiber – 4g
- Sugars – 13g
- Protein – 1g

Krill:

- A shrimp-like marine invertebrate.
- Strong source of omega-3.
- A Norwegian word meaning "young fry of fish."
- Feeds upon plankton and is food for other fish.
- Provides protection for a healthy heart, joints and other body systems.
- Studies indicate anti-aging benefits even greater than with Vitamin A & E.
- Eases PMS symptoms.
- Demonstrates anti-aging characteristics such as anti-wrinkling.
- Provides increased energy. Promotes healthy joints.
- Krill provides 48 times more Oxygen Radical Absorbency Capacity than fish oil and 34 times more than Coenzyme Q10.
- Helps boost the immune system. Provides UVA sun blocking capabilities. Improves digestion.
- Increases brain function and concentration.
- Protects cell membrane.

Kudzu Extract:

- Kudzu is a group of plants in the genus Pueraria, in the pea family. They are climbing, coiling, and trailing perennial vines native to much of eastern Asia, southeast Asia, and some Pacific Islands
- Japanese Arrowroot (Pueraria Lobata).
- Good for minor digestive problems.
- May relieve pain and relax muscle spasms.
- Aids in suppressing the desire for alcohol.
- Source of the chemical daidzin or daidzein.
- Helps suppress the appetite.

L-Arginine:

- **Is an amino acid and is considered a Power Nutrient**.
- Can retard tumors.
- Potent antioxidant.
- Retards LDL cholesterol from oxidizing.
- Factors in increasing lean muscle mass and bone density.
- Aids the immune system in decreasing and destroying bacteria, virus, and cancer cells.
- Increases sperm count.
- Increases blood flow to the pelvic regions promoting a boost in sexual readiness in both males or females.
- Needed for formation of protein.

- Key factor in helping the body release the Human Growth Hormone (HOH)
- Helps decrease body fat.
- Prevents and promotes healing of hemorrhoids and anal fissures by relaxing the hypertonic sphincter muscles.
- Helps in lung disorders by allowing easier breathing.
- Is body's chief source for creating nitric oxide.
- Reduces healing time of injuries (especially bones).
- Helps improve insulin sensitivity.
- Relaxes and dilates the arteries, helping to normalize high blood pressure.
- Is a strong vasodilator.
- Is a powerful anticoagulant that helps the blood from clumping together thereby preventing possible heart attacks, strokes, and angina pain.
- Increases blood flow to the brain thus helping with Alzheimer disease and memory loss.
- Aids the body by allowing more oxygen and nutrition to get to cells through vasodilation.

L-Carnitine:

- It is biosynthesized from amino acids

lysine and methionine.

- Aids in weight loss.
- Decreases risk heart disease.
- Improves athletic ability.
- Helps to transport long-chain fatty acids.

L-Citrulline:

- **Is an amino acid and is considered a Power Nutrient**.
- An amino acid required for detoxification of the liver from ammonia.
- Promotes energy.
- Increases recovery time from exhaustion.
- Helps the immune system function.
- Helps to form L-Arginine through a series of metabolic actions.
- Helps increase and sustain the level of nitric oxide in the blood.
- Useful in building muscle during body building exercise.

L-Cysteine:

- **Is an amino acid and is considered a Power Nutrient.**
- Amino acid with high sulfur content.
- Helps eliminate toxins.
- Free radical destroyer.
- Breaks down mucus.
- Muscle builder.

L-Glutamine:

- **Is an amino acid and is considered a Power Nutrient**.
- Helps with cravings, especially for alcoholism and/or sugar.
- Important for mental ability.
- Prevents schizophrenia and mental retardation.
- Helps with epilepsy, fatigue and impotence.

L-Phenylalanine:

- **Is an amino acid and is considered a Power Nutrient**.
- Amino acid which produces neurotransmitters, therefore, aids in memory and learning.
- Reduces hunger.
- Decreases pain.

L-Taurine:

- **Is an amino acid and is considered a Power Nutrient**.
- Necessary for healthy eyes.
- Good antioxidant.

Lactobacillus Acidophilus:

- "Friendly" bacteria in the intestinal tract that greatly aids in the digestion of protein and inhibits pathogenic organisms.
- Taking a good probiotic on a regular basis will greatly enhance the availability of this bacteria.
- Increases the absorption of all nutrients.
- Fights cancer.
- Helps ear problems.
- Helps skin problems.
- Anti-inflammatory for mucous membranes.
- Increases milk supply for nursing mothers.
- Helps regulate hormones.
- Aids in constipation.
- Calcium metabolism strengthens connective tissue.

Lactobacillus Sporogenes:

- Helps create healthy intestinal bacteria (flora).
- Activated in stomach and goes to small intestine.
- Helps maintain healthy digestion.

Lecithin:

- Fatty nutrient mainly composed of

Vitamin B (Choline).

- Available from sources such as soybeans, eggs, marine sources, etc.
- Effects the permeability of cell membranes which regulates what may enter or leave the cell.
- Promotes energy and is a natural fat emulsifier.
- All living cell membranes are composed of lecithin.

Leeks:

- Good amounts of soluble and insoluble fiber.
- Helps with cholesterol control.
- Has anti-bacterial, anti-viral and anti-fungal activities.
- Good source of vitamin A.

Lemon:

- Rich in dietary fiber.
- Excellent source of vitamin C.
- Phytochemical that improves immune system.
- Good source of vitamin A.
- Helps prevents some cancers.
- Nutritional Facts:
  - Serving Size – 2.1 oz.
  - Calories – 15
  - Fat – 0g

- Dietary Fiber – 2g
- Sugars – 0g
- Protein – 0g

Lemon Balm (Extract):

- Flavonoids and polyphenolics may help with herpes simplex and with hyperthyroidism (Grave's disease).
- May help with flatulence.
- Used for insomnia.
- Helps with nerve pain.
- Antiviral and antibacterial effects.
- Known for helping depression.

Lemon Bioflavonoid:

- Therapeutic for those on a high fat/protein diet.
- Destroys putrefactive bacteria in intestines and mouth.
- Useful during dysentery, colds, flu, hacking coughs, parasite infestation.

Lemon Pectin:

- Used for varicose veins and hemorrhoids, bronchial congestion & kidney stones.
- Has anti-inflammatory and diuretic properties.
- May improve circulation in extremities.

Lemongrass:

- Primary chemical component citral has anti-microbial and anti-fungal properties.
- Essential oils have anti-septic properties.
- Good amount of folic acid.
- Rich in essential vitamins.

Lettuce:

- Rich source of vitamin A, K and B-complex and good source of vitamin C and folates.
- Nutritional Facts:
  - Serving Size – 3.0oz.
  - Calories – 15
  - Fat – 0 g
  - Dietary Fiber – 1 g
  - Sugars – 1g
  - Protein – 1 g

Lettuce, Wild:

- Contains amino acids, minerals, and vitamins.
- Useful for insomnia because of lactucin.
- Useful in alleviating restlessness and excitability (especially in children).
- Used for dysmennhorea.

- Used for coughs.
- Improves circulation, decreases cholesterol.
- Helps to reduce blood sugar.
- Contains carminative properties which help with flatulence and bloating.

Licorice (Root):

- Detoxifies blood.
- Natural sweetener for diabetics.
- Stimulates natural production of cortisone.
- Balances adrenal system.
- Excellent for stress, hypoglycemia, ulcers .
- Estrogen "like" effect on body.
- Helps with herpes, hepatitis, HIV/AIDS, flu, measles.
- Immune enhancer.
- Helps with chronic fatigue syndrome, Chron's disease, ulcers, Lyme disease.
- Can help to fight cancer toxins including chemotherapy toxins.

Limonene:

- An essential oil found in the peel of oranges and lemons.

Lutein:

- **Is an antioxidant which is considered a Power Nutrient.**
- A carotenoid.
- When deposited in the eye reduces risk of macular degeneration and cataracts.
- Reduces oxidation.
- Available in spinach, kale, collard greens, and marigold petals.

Lycopene:

- Bright
  red carotene and carotenoid pigment
  and phytochemical found in tomatoes and other red fruits and vegetables.
- Protects against prostate cancer.
- Lowers risk of cervical and intestinal cancers.

Lysine:

- **Is an amino acid and is considered a Power Nutrient**.
- Plays a major role in calcium absorption.
- Helps building muscle protein.
- Recovery from surgery or sports injuries.
- Helps the body's production of hormones, enzymes and antibodies.
- Highly beneficial to those with herpes simples infections.

- Recommended supplementation of 1,000 to 2,000 mg daily for immune enhancement.

Maca:

- **Is considered a super food.**
- Hearty root vegetable grows in the high Andean plateaus of Peru.
- Full of essential nutrients.
- Positive support for hormonal issues.
- Promotes reproductive health.
- Enhances fertility in both men and women.
- Alleviates minor discomforts symptoms of menopause and PMS.
- Supports normal bone retention during menopause.
- Boosts energy levels and aids in athletic performance.
- Helps strengthen immune system.
- Promotes mental clarity.
- Increases resistance to stress, trauma, anxiety and fatigue.
- Helps maintain normal cholesterol levels.

Macadamia nuts:

- Packed with numerous health-benefiting nutrient, minerals, antioxidants and vitamins that are essential for optimal

health and wellness.
- Gluten free.
- Rich source of mono-unsaturated fatty acid which offers protection from coronary artery disease and strokes.
- Excellent source of minerals like selenium which is cardio protective.
- Nutritional Facts:
  - Serving Size – 1 oz.
  - Calories – 204
  - Dietary Fiber – 2.4 g
  - Protein – 2.2 g

Mace spice:

- Good source of vitamin A and C.
- Has many essential volatile oils.
- Good amount of calcium and iron.

Mackerel:

- **Brain booster**.
- Cold water fish.
- Good source of EPA and DHA
- Considered to be ecology safe.

Mango:

- Rich in dietary fiber, vitamins, minerals and antioxidants.
- Excellent source of vitamin A.
- Good source of vitamins C, E and B6 and

potassium.

- Helps prevent cancer.
- Helps control heart rate and blood pressure.

Magnesium:

- Vital to enzyme activity and assists in calcium and potassium assimilation.
- Protects the arterial linings from stress, so instrumental in preventing heart disease and high blood pressure.
- Affects nerve and muscle impulses and dizziness.
- Helps avoid depression.
- Oxide form is used as a foaming and anti-caking agent.
- Citrate form is used as a buffer and neutralizer in beverages.

Marine Lipid Complex (Fish Oils):

- Helps to lubricate joints.
- Provides healthy brain cell tissue.
- Found to help children with attention deficit disorder.
- Promotes mental clarity and "good vibrations" (mood).
- Great for the heart (tends to lower cholesterol and promote a healthy inflammation response as measured for C-reactive protein levels).

Marshmallow (Root):

- A perennial herb native to Europe and western Asia.
- Tranquilizing herb.
- Is a blood purifier and diuretic.
- Used commonly in cough medicines and as an eye bath.
- Protects skin and helps in healing wounds.

Medium Chain Triglycerides:

- Medium sized essential fatty acids.
- Useful for athletes.
- Supplies fast source of energy.
- Increases metabolism.
- Helps develop muscles.

Melatonin:

- **Is an antioxidant which is considered a Power Nutrient.**
- Synchronizes hormone secretion.
- Biological time-keeper.
- Cancer preventative.
- Induces sleep.
- Helps reduce insomnia.
- Useful in overcoming jet lag.
- Antidepressant.

Milk, Nonfat:

- Solid part of cow's milk after removing water.
- Contains more protein, vitamins, & minerals per gram than whole milk.

Milk Protein Concentrate:

- Can be a source of protein.
- Used for many purposes in food processing and recipes.
- Form can vary in percentage of protein, minerals, fat, and lactose.

Milk Thistle Extract:

- Consists of chemical called silymarin.
- Factor in the regeneration of liver and gallbladder cells.
- Aids the production of mother's milk.
- Antioxidant.
- Blocks liver poisons.
- Removes toxins from the liver.
- May help with psoriasis.
- Reduces cholesterol levels in bile which may help prevent gallstones.

Mixed Carotene (Vitamin A):

- **Is an antioxidant which is considered a Power Nutrient**.

- Slows aging.
- Enhances immunity by protecting mucous membranes.
- Prevents night blindness and other eye problems.
- Great for skin disorders.
- Utilizes protein.
- Key in formulation of bones and teeth.
- Enhances growth and repair of body tissue.

Mixed Tocopherols:

- **Is an antioxidant which is considered a Power Nutrient**.
- Sometimes added to protect flavor.
- Key to cellular respiration.
- Prevents cell damage and repairs tissue while reducing scarring.
- Critical to the normal clotting of the blood.
- Strengthens capillary walls and produces red blood cells.
- Seems to have a dramatic effect on the reproductive system of both males and females.
- Can be a diuretic to the system.

Molybdenum:

- Critical to the oxidation of fats and irons.

- Enables body to use nitrogen and converts purines to uric acid.
- Good for sexual impotence in males over 45.
- May suppress tumors.
- Mineral attached to protein molecule to transport it to the blood stream in order to enhance its absorption.

Mononitrate (Thiamin):

- Synthetic form of Vitamin B1.
- Promotes growth.
- Aids digestion, especially of carbohydrates.
- Improves mental attitude.
- Fights against air or sea sickness.
- Helps treat Herpes.
- Fights against Beriberi disease.

Moringa:

- **Is considered a super food**.
- Moringa is a genus of trees indigenous to Southern India and Northern Africa. Now cultivated in Central and South America, etc.
- Leaves are a healthy aging powerhouse contain powerful nutrient zeatin.
- Helps slow abnormal cell growth.

Mulberries:

- Excellent source of vitamin C
- Rich in some phytochemicals that protect against cancer, aging and neurological diseases, inflammation, diabetes and bacterial infections.
- Rich in B-complex and vitamin K.
- Excellent source of iron which determines the oxygen-carrying capacity of the blood.

Mushroom Extract, Dried Reishi:

- Studies show Reishi to be helpful with high blood pressure, high triglycerides, and cancer.
- Used by Chinese to treat fatigue, asthma, insomnia, high cholesterol, and viral infections.
- Promotes the digestion of infectious bacteria such as yeast and bronchial infections.
- Helps to prevent cirrhosis of the liver and fatty liver from alcoholism.
- Helps to fight against various cancers, especially liver cancer.
- It has been found to lower pain and decrease stress.
- **Caution: Use under a doctor's care if taking blood thinning medications.

Mushroom, Shiitake (Whole):

- Contains a potent anti-cancer and antiviral.
- Effective in heart disease by lowering cholesterol and blood pressure.
- Is an antiviral and overcomes fatigue while increasing cell longevity.
- Valuable to fight LNKS, chronic fatigue syndrome, and Lyme disease.
- Stimulates the immune system to fight a variety of problems including the above and colds.
- **Caution: Rare reactions such as hives and diarrhea. Has good record of safety.
- Nutritional Facts:
    - Serving Size – 3.0oz.
    - Calories – 20
    - Fat – 0 g
    - Dietary Fiber – 1 g
    - Sugars – 0g
    - Protein – 3 g

Mustard:

- Source of major antioxidant *isothiocyanates*.
- **Antioxidants are considered a Power Nutrient.**

Mustard greens:

- Storehouse of many phyto-nutrients.

- Good amount of fiber.
- High in vitamin K and good source of vitamin A, C and folic acid.
- Helps prevent various cancers.

Mustard seeds:

- High in essential oils as well as plant sterols.
- Excellent source of essential B-complex vitamins.
- Contain flavonoid and carotenoid antioxidants.

N-Acetyl Cysteine:

- A nutritional supplement.
- Used to promote wound healing.
- Used to decrease side effects of chemotherapy and radiation therapy.
- May prevent aging by increasing levels of the potent antioxidant, glutathione.

Natural Caffeine:

- Stimulating ingredient.
- Enhances fat oxidation by increasing circulating fatty acids.

Neptune Krill Oil (NKO®):

- Oil derived from shrimp-like marine invertebrate.

- The word "Krill" comes from the Norwegian word meaning "young fry of fish".
- Provides protection for a healthy heart, joints and other body systems.
- Studies indicate anti-aging benefits even greater than with Vitamin A & E.
- Eases PMS symptoms.
- Demonstrates anti-aging characteristics such as anti-wrinkling.
- Provides increased energy.
- Promotes healthy joints.
- Krill provides 48 times more Oxygen Radical Absorbency Capacity than fish oil and 34 times more than Coenzyme QlO.
- Helps boost the immune system.
- Provides UVA sun blocking capabilities.
- Improves digestion.
- Increases brain function and concentration.
- Protects cell membrane.

Nettle Extract:
- Promotes colon health.
- Aids urinary problems.
- Helpful with arthritis.
- Assists hemorrhoid healing.
- Good for cystitis, worms, asthma, and eczema.
- Helpful with diarrhea, nephritis.

- Pain reliever and expectorant.
- Good for inflammatory conditions.

Niacin (Vitamin B3):

- Helps schizophrenia.
- Lowers cholesterol.
- Promotes healthy skin.
- Aids the nervous system.
- Helps metabolize carbohydrates, fats, and proteins.
- Aids digestion.

Nitric Oxide (NO):

Nitric Oxide is a naturally occurring chemical that has many functions in the body. Nitric oxide is essential for the promotion of both your health and longevity. The cardiovascular system uses NO to control blood flow to every part of the body. NO improves blood flow, thereby increasing oxygen delivery to tissues and removing waste products at the same time. This is critical in order to maintain normal organ function it is also critical for maintaining maximal muscle performance during exercise. This is how NO acts as a signaling molecule to promote cellular nutrition. NO is the body's most important molecule for promoting cellular nutrition.

- Lowers the blood pressure and protects against hypertension

- Prevents unwanted blood clotting
- Lowers bad cholesterol (LDL)
- Protects against vascular complications of diabetes
- Protects against early stages of Alzheimer's disease
- Protects against gastrointestinal ulcers
- Protects against urinary incontinence in women
- Protects against oxidative stress-mediated tissue injury such as inflammation and arthritis
- Functions as the neurotransmitter that stimulates erectile function in both men and women
- Enhances physical performance, shortens recovery and increase endurance during exercise.

The body's production of NO lowers with age and thus supplementation is required. Niteworks has been developed Dr. Louis Ignarro, Ph.D. won the 1998 Nobel Prize in Medicine for his work on NO. It can be found at my product store at: http://herbal-nutrition.net/rodstone.

Notoginseng Extract, Dried Panax:

- Notoginseng belongs to the same scientific genus as Asian ginseng. It grows naturally

in China and Japan.
- Improves endurance.
- Improves memory and mental function.
- Stimulates adrenal glands, pancreas, and pituitary gland.
- Lowers blood sugar.
- Reduces inflammation.

Nutmeg:

- Good source of minerals like copper and potassium.
- Rich in many vital B-complex vitamins.
- Contains many essential volatiles oils.

Oat Fiber:

- Source of fiber that lowers cholesterol significantly.

Oats:

- **Heart smart food**.
- Whole grain with lots of fiber.
- Lowers cholesterol because of fiber.
- Good source of minerals and Vitamins E & Bs.
- No gluten.
- Has both soluble and insoluble fiber.
- Aids constipation.
- Nutritional Facts:
  - Serving Size – 100 g.

- Calories –389
- Dietary Fiber – 10.6 g
- Protein – 16.9 g

Oligofructose:

- A non-digestible fructo-oligosaccharide.
- Referred to as FOS.
- Occurs naturally in a variety of fruits, vegetables, and grains.
- Shown to inhibit malignant tumor growth.
- Can help promote up to a ten-fold increase in the growth of bifidobacteria.

Okra:

- Rich in dietary fiber.
- Healthy amounts of vitamin A and K.
- Rich in vitamin C and B-complex.
- Helps reduce episodes of cold and cough.
- Prevents some cancers.

Olive:

- Contain significant amounts of plant-derived antioxidants, minerals, phyto-sterols and vitamins.
- Help to prevent coronary artery disease and strokes.
- Contains compounds that play a vital role fighting against cancer, inflammation, coronary artery disease, degenerative

nerve diseases, diabetes, etc.

Olive Oil:

- **Heart smart food.**
- **Brain booster**.
- Useful as a cooking oil.
- Lowers LDL, bad cholesterol and raises HDL, good cholesterol.
- A mono unsaturated fat better for the heart.
- Tends to lower the formation of gallstones.
- Protects the stomach to discourage ulcers and gastritis.
- Strong antioxidant properties, especially Vitamin E.
- Studies show it may lower the risk of colon cancer

Omega-3 Fatty Acids – EPA, DHA and ALA

- **Is considered a Power Nutrient**.
- 80% of the population does not get enough.
- Our bodies cannot make the three most important types of essential fatty acids, EPA (eicosapentaenoic acid), DHA (docosahexaenoic acid) and ALA (alpha-linolenic acid) – so we must get them

from our diets or supplementation.

- ALA is found in vegetables sources like flaxseed, but it does not have the same potent health benefits as EPA and DHA.
- EPA and DHA are found in marine sources and have the common name, "fish oil."
- Two types of omega fatty acids dominate our foods: Omega—3 from marine sources, grasses, etc. and Omega −6 from grains. It is suggested to have a ratio of Omega − 6 to Omega − 3 of 1:1 to 4:1. However, the typical America diet is 14:1 to 30:1 or higher.
- Is an anti-inflammatory.
- Antioxidant
- Stave off cardiovascular disease.
- Can help lower triglycerides and apoproteins which are markers of diabetes.
- Helps with weight control and fitness.
- By lowering inflammation it helps with arthritis.
- Helps with bone density so lowers osteoporosis.
- Has been shown to help control mental illness.
- Shown to help with Attention Deficit Hyperactivity Disorder (ADHD).
- Recommended Supplementation: maintenance of optimal health − 500 − 3,000 mg per day. Obesity, diabetes,

cardiovascular dysfunction and other enhanced health concerns – 1,500 – 9,00 mg per day.

Onion:

- **Heart smart food**.
- Rich in soluble dietary fiber.
- Rich in phyto-chemicals.
- Good in B-complex.
- Helps control cholesterol.
- Protects from cancers.
- Helps control blood sugar levels.
- Found to have anti-carcinogenic, anti-inflammatory and anti-diabetic functions
- Nutritional Facts:
  - Serving Size – 5.3 oz.
  - Calories – 45
  - Fat – 0 g
  - Dietary Fiber – 3 g
  - Sugars – 9g
  - Protein – 1 g

Onion, Dried Green:

- Used for flavoring.
- Boosts friendly bacteria and immune system.
- Contains sulfides known to lower blood pressure and blood lipids.
- Onions in general have an anti-tumor effect.
- Study indicated decrease in stomach cancer when large quantities of onions

were consumed.

- Uncontrolled studies showed onions can lower sugar levels in diabetes.
- Other studies show that onions may help with asthma, eczema, coughs and infections.

Onion Powder:

- Often used as a flavoring.
- Works against infection
- Lowers blood pressure
- Reduces blood sugar levels.
- Helps with spasms.
- Relaxes spasms.
- May increase HDL while lowering LDL.
- Reduces blood clotting substances which helps lower the risk of stroke.
- Source of Vitamin C.

Orange:

- **Heart smart food**.
- Nutrients in oranges are plentiful and diverse.
- Excellent source of vitamin C.
- Good source of vitamin A and B-complex and other flavonoid antioxidants.
- Helps the immune system.
- Control heart rate and blood pressure.
- Rich in dietary fiber.

- Helps control cholesterol.
- Helps prevent some cancers.
- Nutritional Facts:
  - Serving Size – 5.5 oz.
  - Calories – 80
  - Fat – 0g
  - Dietary Fiber – 3g
  - Sugars – 14
  - Protein – 1g

Orange Fruit Bioflavonoids:

- A group of phytochemicals that work with Vitamin C to keep the body healthy, reduce the risk of cancer, strengthen bones and teeth, help heal wounds, keep skin healthy, and lower the risk of heart attack.
- Bioflavonoids and Vitamin C are powerful antioxidants working as a team which help protect the body from free radicals. It's important to get them from whole foods such as orange- and yellow-colored fruits and vegetables.
- Previously known as Vitamin P collectively, these bioflavonoids include a number of Vitamin C-like components that work together with citrin, rutin, flavonol, catechin , proanthocyanidins, poly phenols and quercetin.
- Have antiviral, anti-cancer and anti-allergic actions.
- Helpful in the absorption of Vitamin C.
- Improves and prolongs the function of

Vitamin C.

- Indirectly involved in maintaining the health of collagen which holds the tissues of the body together in bone, teeth, and scars formed during wound healing and bone fractures.
- The anti-inflammatory and collagen repair action of bioflavonoids may help joint and connective tissue problems such as tendinitis, arthritis, rheumatoid arthritis, injury, fibromyalgia and gout.
- Main function is to increase the strength of the capillaries.
- By supporting the capillaries they help to prevent hemorrhage and rupture of tiny vessels which could lead to bruising, bleeding gums, and duodenal bleeding ulcers.
- May be helpful in the maintenance of capillary health and reduction of bleeding in such conditions as hemorrhoids, varicose veins, spontaneous abortions, excessive menstrual bleeding and chronic nose bleeds.
- High intake of bioflavonoids has been linked to a lower risk of heart attack.
- Contributes to Vitamin C applications such as treatment of cold and flu.
- Bioflavonoids have been useful in asthma, allergies, bursitis and arthritis, eye problems secondary to diabetes, and as protection from the harmful effects of

radiation.

Orange Peel (Citrus Aurantium) (Peel):

- Relieves tension.
- Relaxes spasms.
- Improves digestion.
- Useful in treating colic and stress.

Orange Pekoe:

- "Orange" is used as a descriptive word referring to the size of the leaf.
- Made from the same leaves as green tea.
- Allowed to ferment and age longer than green tea.
- The fermentation process gives a deeper richer flavor but may destroy some of the active and/or beneficial components.
- Contains more caffeine than Green Tea.
- Provides energy.

Oregano:

- Essential oils anti-septic, anti-spasmodic, carminative, cholagogue, diaphoretic, expectorant, stimulant and mildly tonic properties.
- Taken for treatment of colds, influenza, mild fevers, indigestion, stomach upsets and painful menstruation conditions.
- Has anti-bacterial and anti-fungal

activities.
- Rich in antioxidants like vitamin A and C.
- Excellent source of minerals like potassium.

Oriental Ginseng Extract, Dried:

- King of tonics.
- Stimulates entire body energy.
- Cardiovascular regulator and stimulant.

Ornithine Alpha-Ketoglutarate:

- Nutritional supplement.
- Releases growth hormone that metabolizes excess body fat when combined with L-arginine and L-carnitine.
- Necessary for immune system and liver function.
- Helps body process urea and citric acid.
- Aids the body in the breakdown of food.

Panax Ginseng (Root):

- Asian Ginseng.
- Studies indicate ginseng is helpful with erectile dysfunction.
- May be helpful with epilepsy.
- Increases general sense of well-being.
- Increases mental & physical activity.
- Enhances immune functions.
- May help with blood glucose levels in type

2 diabetes.

Pantothenic Acid (Vitamin B5):

- Pantothen is Greek meaning everywhere. Small quantities of pantothenic acid are found in nearly every food.
- Critical to cell metabolism.
- Is activating agent.
- Releases energy from carbohydrates, fats, and proteins.
- Increases production of cortisone, steroids, and antibodies.
- Reduces toxic effects of antibiotics.
- Wonderful aid in healing wounds.
- Fights infection.
- Helps prevent fatigue.
- Good for hypoglycemia, ulcers, and blood and skin disorders.

Papaya:

- Good source of soluble fiber.
- Rich in vitamin A, C, and B-complex.
- Good amount of potassium.
- Immune booster and anti-inflammatory.
- Protect the body from lung and oral cavity cancers.

Parsley:

- Essential oil found to reduce blood sugar

levels in diabetics.
- Rich in flavonoid antioxidants.
- Good source of minerals like potassium which helps control heart rate and blood pressure.
- Rich in antioxidant vitamins A, C, E, etc.
- Richest of the entire herb source for vitamin K.

Parsnips:

- Excellent source of soluble and insoluble dietary fiber.
- Rich in B-complex.
- Good amount of vitamin C.

Peach:

- Good source of vitamin A, C, and B-carotene.
- Rich in potassium and other vital minerals.
- Helps prevent from lung and oral cavity cancers.
- Helps regulate the heart rate and blood pressure.
- Nutritional Facts:
  - Serving Size – 5.3 oz.
  - Calories – 60
  - Fat – 0g
  - Dietary Fiber – 2 g
  - Sugars – 13 g
  - Protein – 1 g

Peanuts:

- Heart smart food.
- Good source of protein.
- Excellent source of resveratrol which protects against cancers, heart disease, degenerative nerve disease, Alzheimer's disease, and viral/fungal infections.
- Excellent source of vitamin E and B-complex.
- Nutritional Facts:
  - Serving Size – 1 oz.
  - Calories –166
  - Dietary Fiber – 6.7 g
  - Protein – 2.3 g

Pear:

- Rich in dietary fiber.
- Good in vitamin A and C.
- Helps regulate cholesterol levels.
- Helps with weight management.
- Nutritional Facts:
  - Serving Size – 5.9 oz.
  - Calories – 100
  - Fat – 0g
  - Dietary Fiber – 6 g
  - Sugars – 16 g
  - Protein – 1 g

Peas:

- Excellent source of folic acid.
- Good amounts of ascorbic acid, vitamin K and A.

Pecans:

- Rich in monounsaturated fatty acids which help to prevent coronary artery disease and strokes.
- Rich source of many phyto-chemical substances that protect from diseases, cancers, as well as infections.
- Excellent source of vitamin E and B-complex.
- Nutritional Facts:
  - Serving Size – 1 oz.
  - Calories –196
  - Dietary Fiber – 2.7 g
  - Protein – 2.6 g

Peppermint:

- Compounds helps with treatment of irritable bowel syndrome and other colic pain disorders.
- Excellent source of minerals like potassium.
- Rich in antioxidant vitamins A, C, E and K.

Phytonadione (Vitamin K):

- Used as an anticoagulant.

- A form of Vitamin K used as a supplement to prevent bleeding disorders.

Phytosterol Esters:

- Natural substances found in soybeans, corn, and other plants.
- Studies indicate a decrease in LDL cholesterol and reduction of plaque formation.
- The American diet consists of about 80 mg of phytosterol esters daily a stark contrast to a vegetarian or Japanese diet which contains 345 - 400 mg per day.

Pine nuts:

- Rich in monounsaturated fatty acids that help prevent coronary artery disease and strokes.
- Contain essential fatty acid that helps with weight loss.
- Excellent source of vitamin E and B-complex.
- Gluten free.
- Nutritional Facts:
  - Serving Size – 1 oz.
  - Calories –191
  - Dietary Fiber – 1.0 g
  - Protein – 3.8 g

Pine Bark Extract, (Pycnogenol®) :

- Pycnogenol® is a branded antioxidant which is manufactured from French maritime pine bark, touted as a natural botanical antioxidant.
- Has the unique ability to cross the blood / brain barrier to protect the brain and nerve tissue from oxidation.
- Allows for improved cellular nutrition.
- Anti-inflammatory.
- Produces immunomodulation.
- Offsets the constriction of blood vessels.
- Has vascular relaxant properties working with nitric oxide.
- Helps to balance LDL and HDL for healthier cholesterol.

Pineapple:
- Excellent source of vitamin C and B-complex.
- Boost immunity and pro-inflammatory.
- Helps protect against some cancers.
- Helps fight against arthritis and indigestion.
- Nutritional Facts:
    - Serving Size – 4 oz.
    - Calories – 50
    - Fat – 0g
    - Dietary Fiber – 1 g
    - Sugars – 10 g
    - Protein – 1 g

Pistachio nuts:

- Rich in monounsaturated fatty acids which help to prevent coronary artery disease and strokes.
- Rich in phyto-chemical substances which help protect the body from diseases, cancers, as well as infections.
- Excellent source of vitamin E and B-complex.
- Excellent source or minerals that help with neuro-transmission, metabolism as well as red blood cell synthesis.
- Nutritional Facts:
    - Serving Size – 1 oz.
    - Calories –162
    - Dietary Fiber – 2.9 g
    - Protein – 6.0 g

Plums:

- Good source of vitamin A and C.
- Helps the digestive system.
- Helps prevent some cancers.
- Controls heart rate and blood pressure.
- Nutritional Facts:
    - Serving Size – 5.4 oz.
    - Calories – 70
    - Fat – 0g
    - Dietary Fiber – 2 g
    - Sugars – 16 g
    - Protein – 1 g

Pomegranate:

- **Pomegranate is considered a Power Nutrient**.
- In ancient Greek mythology, the pomegranate represents life and regeneration.
- Pomegranate juice contains a higher level of polyphenol antioxidants than red wine, cranberry juice cocktail and blueberry juice.
- Protects and enhances the functions and benefits of nitric oxide (NO) in the cardiovascular system.
- Rich source of soluble and insoluble dietary fibers.
- Antioxidant protection.
- Treatment of cardiovascular dysfunction, diabetes, metabolic syndrome and obesity
- Osteoarthritis treatment.
- Erectile dysfunction treatment.
- Immune support.
- Alzheimer's disease prevention.
- Controls cholesterol.
- Improves blood pressure.
- Protects against various cancers.
- Recommended supplementation: 8 to 16 ounces of juice per day. Natural pomegranate polyphenol extract – 1,000 mg per day.

Poppy seeds:

- Good source of dietary fiber.
- Rich in monounsaturated fatty acid which helps to prevent coronary artery disease and strokes.
- Excellent source of B-complex.
- Good source of minerals which help with digestion, nucleic acid syntheses, controlling heart rate and blood pressure.

Potassium:

- Critical to healthy cardiovascular functioning.
- Stabilizes blood pressure, regulates heart rhythm.
- Affects health of nervous system and muscle contractions.
- Regulates water balance and alkalinity of body fluids as well as the transfer of nutrients to cells.
- Flavor enhancer agent, gelling agent, and salt substitute.

Potato:

- Rich in dietary fiber.
- Rich in B-complex.
- Nutritional Facts:
  - Serving Size – 5.3 oz.
  - Calories – 110
  - Fat – 0 g

- Dietary Fiber – 2 g
- Sugars – 1 g
- Protein – 3 g

Powdered Cellulose:

- Supplement.
- Powdered form of cellulose or fiber which is essential to the smooth functioning of the large bowel.

Propylparaben:

- Propylparaben occurs as a natural substance found in many plants and some insects, although it is manufactured synthetically for use in cosmetics, pharmaceuticals and foods.
- Preservative.
- Anti-fungal and anti-bacterial agent.

Protein, Isolated Soy:

- Provides most of the essential amino acids.
- No cholesterol.
- Low in fat.
- Has isoflavones which are antioxidants and may help with menopause symptoms.
- May reduce the risk of hormone dependent cancers.
- Provides genistein and daidzein.
- Promotes healthy blood serum

cholesterol.

Psyllium Seed Husk:

- Psyllium seed husk are portions of the seeds of the plant Plantago ovata a native of India and Pakistan.
- Source of soluble dietary fiber.
- Fiber which cleans the intestines by absorbing water and expanding many times in size.
- Softens stools and helps body avoid colitis and constipation.

Pumpkin:

- Rich in vitamin A, C and E.
- Good so B-complex.
- Anti-oxidant prevents age related macular disease.

Pumpkin Seed:

- Rich in monounsaturated fatty acids to help prevent coronary artery disease and strokes.
- Excellent source of amino acids that convert to serotonin, (nature's sleeping pill).
- Anti-stress.
- Used to support the prostate.
- Rich in zinc.

- Nutritional Facts:
  - Serving Size – 1 oz.
  - Calories –163
  - Dietary Fiber – 1.8 g
  - Protein – 8.5 g

Pumpkin Seed Powder:

- Supplies generous amounts of oil, vitamins, and minerals.
- Excellent source of iron.
- Good source of zinc.
- Inhibits bone loss.
- Keeps collagen healthy.
- Increases strength and permeability of the capillaries.
- Helps lower cholesterol.

Pyridoxal 5 - Phosphate & Pyridoxine Hydrochloride (Vitamin B$_6$):

- Involved in more body functions than any other single nutrient.
- Essential to synthesis of RNA, DNA, and, therefore, directly affects the reproduction and growth of all cells.
- Helps in absorption of fats and proteins as well as in the stimulation of proper digestive juices, so is critical in the weight loss process.
- Aids in production of digestive juices.
- Red blood cells coenzyme and antibody

formulator.
- Maintains balance of sodium and potassium.
- Insures the smooth functioning of both the immune and nervous systems.
- Necessary for production of hydrochloric acid.
- Decreases symptoms of P.M.S.
- Helps with allergies, arthritis, and asthma.
- Been known to help carpal tunnel syndrome.
- Helps heart by reducing cholesterol around it.
- Enhances the immune system.
- Aids production of antibodies.

Quercetin:

- A flavonoid found in fruits, vegetables, leaves and grains.
- Also available as part of supplement.
- Potent inhibitor of cancer cell growth.
- May stop the onset of mammary tumors.
- Inhibits the growth of breast cancer cells.
- Potent antioxidant inhibiting LDL oxidation.
- A strong antioxidant that destroys damaging free radicals.
- Protects the heart and may counter some of the damaging effects following a heart

attack.

- Appears to lower high blood pressure.
- Works in conjunction with the process of metabolizing fat.
- Work to balance the energizing effects of caffeine.
- Used extensively in athletic injuries.
- Enhances absorption of Vitamin C.
- May decrease allergic reactions.
- Offsets the constriction of blood vessels.
- Has vascular relaxant properties working with nitric oxide.
- Helps to balance LDL and HDL for healthier cholesterol.

Quinoa:

- Good source of high quality protein.
- Gluten-free.
- Rich source of soluble and insoluble fiber.
- Excellent source of vitamin A, B-compex and many antioxidants.
- Helps protect from cancers, infection, against and degenerative neurological diseases.
- Antiseptic.
- Nutritional Facts:
  - Serving Size – 100 g
  - Calories –120
  - Dietary Fiber – 2.8 g
  - Protein – 4.4 g

Quinquefolius Extract, Dried Panax (Root):
- American Ginseng.
- Useful in fighting fatigue and stress.
- May be helpful with diabetes.
- Useful in sexual dysfunction.
- Improves athletic performance.

Radishes:
- Source of major antioxidant *isothiocyanates*.
- Prevention of prostate, breast, colon and ovarian cancers.
- Rich in vitamin C.
- Nutritional Facts:
  - Serving Size – 3.0 oz.
  - Calories – 10
  - Fat – 0 g
  - Dietary Fiber – 1 g
  - Sugars – 2 g
  - Protein – 0 g

Raspberries:
- Excellent source of vitamin C.
- Good source of vitamin A and E.
- Contains antioxidants that protects against cancer, aging, inflammation and

neuro-degenerative diseases.
- Helps control heart rate and blood pressure.

Red Clover:

- Wonderful for scrofulous and skin diseases.
- Great antidote for cancer.
- Helps bronchitis, leprosy, syphilis, rickets, indolent ulcers.

Red Clover Extract:

- Used as a blood purifier.
- Has antispasmodic properties.
- Makes a good sedative to relax muscle cramping and nervous exhaustion.
- Relieves irritation and inflammation of the urinary tract.
- Used for menopausal problems.

Reishi Mushroom Extract, Dried:

- Studies show Reishi to be helpful with high blood pressure, high triglycerides, and cancer.
- Used by Chinese to treat fatigue, asthma, insomnia, high cholesterol, and viral infections.

- Promotes the digestion of infectious bacteria such as yeast and bronchial infections.
- Helps to prevent cirrhosis of the liver and fatty liver from alcoholism.
- Helps to fight against various cancers, especially liver cancer.
- It has been found to lower pain and decrease stress.
- **Caution: Use under a doctor's care if taking blood thinning medications.

Resveratrol:

- **Is an antioxidant which is considered a Power Nutrient**
- Is an antioxidant produced by several plants like the skin of red grapes.
- An especially potent antioxidant.
- It helps lower the chances of coronary heart disease.

Retinyl Acetate 50% and Beta Carotene 50% (Vitamin A):

- Antioxidant.
- Slows aging.
- Enhances immunity by protecting mucous membranes.
- Prevents night blindness and other eye problems.
- Great for skin disorders.

- Utilizes protein.
- Key in the formulation of bones and teeth.
- Enhances growth and repair of body tissue.

Rhodiola Extract, Dried (Root):

- Called Rhodiola Rosea.
- A cardio protector.
- Used for depression.
- Alleviates anxiety.
- Works as an anti-inflammatory.
- Remarkable ability to increase resistance to numerous chemical, physical, and biological stresses including strenuous exercise, mental strain, and toxic chemicals.

Rhubarb:

- Contains vitamin A, K and B-complex.
- Prevents some cancers
- Helps in treatment of Alzheimer's.

Riboflavin (Vitamin B2):

- Necessary for cell formation, reproduction, and growth.
- Maintains good vision, nails, hair, and skin.
- Essential in breakdown of carbohydrates,

fats, and proteins.
- Facilitates oxygen use and antibody production.

Ribonucleic Acid (RNA) (Yeast):

- Nucleic acid that transmits to each cell instructions on how to perform.
- Delivers DNA's genetic code to the part of the cell where proteins are manufactured.

Rice:

- **Heart smart food**.
- Rice bran is a proven cholesterol fighter.
- Rich in vitamin E.
- Nutritional Facts:
  - Serving Size – 100 g
  - Calories –112
  - Dietary Fiber – 1.8 g
  - Protein – 2.3 g

Rice Fiber:

- Made from rice hulls and added to some processed foods.
- Digestive tonic.
- Used for bronchial disorders.
- Nutrients and fiber that help curb the appetites.

Rosehips Extract:

- The fruit of the wild rose bush.
- Excellent source of natural Vitamin C.
- Good for stress, bladder problems, and all infections.

Rosemary:

- Rich in B-complex like folic acid.
- Good for vitamin A and C.
- Relaxes spasms.
- Relieves pain.
- Increases perspiration.
- Stimulates the liver.
- Stimulates the gallbladder.
- Improves digestion.
- Controls many pathogenic organisms.
- Helpful with depression, headaches.
- Pregnant woman should take caution.
- Powerful antioxidant with cascading effect.
- Effective at inhibiting carcinogens from damaging cellular DNA.

Rutin:

- Rutin is one of the phenolic compounds found in the invasive plant species *Carpobrotus edulis* and contributes to the antibacterial and antioxidant properties of the plant.

- Used as a dietary supplement for capillary fragility.

Safflower Oil:
- Contains high levels of linoleic or oleic acid and unsaturated fat.
- Helps inflammation in the joints.
- Known to relieve eczema and rough skin.

Saffron:
- Good source of minerals like copper and potassium.
- Rich in many vital vitamins like A, C and folic acid.
- Many essential volatile oils.

Sage:
- Good source of vitamin A and C.
- Benefits in the prevention of cardiovascular diseases.
- Helps dissolve toxins.
- Stimulates hair growth.
- Fights adverse elements that affect the brain.
- Free radical scavenger.
- Helps improve memory.

Salmon:

- **Heart smart food.**
- **Brain booster**.
- Salmon is extra special because it contains Omega −3.
- Helps control cholesterol.
- Nutritional Facts:
    - Serving Size − 3 oz.
    - Calories − 200
    - Fat − 10 g
    - Protein − 24 g

Salt:

- Used as a flavoring.
- Used as a preservative.

Sardines:

- **Brain booster**.
- Found in the coldest waters
- Known to have high levels of EPA and DHA
- Considered to be ecology safe.

Savory:

- Compound carvacrol has anti-bacterial properties.
- Excellent source of minerals and vitamins for optimum health.
- Rich source of B-complex and vitamins A

and C.

Saw Palmetto Lipid Extract:

- Helps with benign prostatic hyperplasia.
- Inhibits inflammatory substances that contribute to prostate problems.

Schizandra:

- A deciduous woody vine native to forest of Northern China and the Russian Far East.
- Known to powerfully increase the immune system functions.
- Protects against stress and increases the energy supply of the cells in the whole body, especially the brain.
- It is a free radical scavenger and normalizes the blood sugar.

Sea Buckthorn:

- Called Hippohae Rharnnoides and grows naturally in the Gobi Desert.
- Rich in Rose Hips Acerola Vitamins A, B12, C & E.
- The berries carry a high content of essential fatty acids.
- The combination of the Vitamin B-12 and Vitamin C work perfectly to enhance metabolic functioning.
- Known and used extensively to maintain healthy skin.

- Protects the healthy mucus of the stomach and acts as an anti-inflammatory.
- Promotes tissue regeneration.
- Helps with stomach ulcers
- Reduces cholesterol.
- Shows anti-cancer activity.
- Inhibits platelet aggregation.

Selenium:

- **Is an antioxidant which is considered a Power Nutrient.**
- Is one of the major antioxidants.
- Stimulates increased antibody process.
- Increases tissue elasticity.
- Works in conjunction with Vitamin E in the promotion of normal body growth and fertility.
- Mineral attaches to protein molecule to transport it to the blood stream in order to enhance its absorption.
- Fights cancer by activating glutathione.
- Recommended supplementation is 200 mcg daily.

Sesame seeds:

- Rich in monounsaturated fatty acid to help prevent coronary artery disease and strokes.
- Good source of protein.

- Good source of many antioxidants.
- Rich in quality vitamins and minerals.
- Helps reduce anxiety and neurosis.
- Rich source of many essential minerals. These help in bone mineralization, red blood cell production, enzyme synthesis, hormone production, as well as regulation of cardiac and skeletal muscle activities.
- Nutritional Facts:
    - Serving Size – 1 T
    - Calories –52
    - Dietary Fiber – 1.1 g
    - Protein – 1.6 g

Shallots:

- Rich in anti-oxidants which have anti-bacterial, anti-viral and anti-fungal activities.
- More concentration of vitamins and minerals than onions.

Shiitake Mushroom:

- Contains a potent anti-cancer and antiviral.
- Effective in heart disease by lowering cholesterol and blood pressure.
- Is an antiviral and overcomes fatigue while increasing cell longevity.
- Valuable to fight LNKS, chronic fatigue syndrome, and Lyme disease.
- Stimulates the immune system to fight a

variety of problems including the above and colds.
- **Caution: Rare reactions such as hives and diarrhea. Has good record of safety.

Short Buchu Extract:

- Originates from South Africa.
- Good for digestion - gas, bloating.
- Is an excellent diuretic and is used for all acute and chronic urinary disorders.
- Fights inflammation of mucous membranes in sinuses due to colds / allergies.
- Aids in controlling diabetes / hypoglycemia.

Silicon Dioxide:

- Has been known since ancient times. Found in nature as quartz as well as in various living organisms.
- Trace mineral necessary for collagen formation and healthy nails, skin, and hair.
- Prevents cardiovascular degeneration by maintaining flexibility in arteries.

Slippery Elm (Bark):

- Helps soothe irritation.
- Aids in dispersing inflammation.

- Assists in rapid healing.
- Great strengthening agent.
- Medicinal uses are: tuberculosis, asthma, bronchitis, pneumonia, gastritis, nephritis, gastric ulcers, ulcerations, calculi (stones or crystals), painful urination, croup, diphtheria, inflammation of the bowels, skin eruptions, sores, ulcerated stomach, stomach weakness, boils, carbuncles, abscesses, wounds, bums, diarrhea, coughs, dysentery, pleurisy, sore throat, poison ivy, female problems, leukorrhea, tumors, vaginal irritation.

Sodium Caseinate:

- An animal protein derived from cow's milk.
- Contains the essential eight amino acids the body cannot manufacture.
- Sodium Caseinate provides a higher nutritional value in supplements.

Sodium Molybdate (Molybdenum):

- Critical to the oxidation of fats and irons.
- Enables body to use nitrogen and converts purines to uric acid.
- Good for sexual impotence in males over 45.

Sodium Selenite:

- **Is an antioxidant which is considered a Power Nutrient.**
- Stimulates increased antibody process.
- Increases tissue elasticity
- Works in conjunction with Vitamin E in the promotion of normal body growth and fertility.
- Mineral attaches to protein molecule to transport it to the blood stream in order to enhance its absorption.

Soy:

- **Heart smart food.**
- Antioxidant.
- May ease menopausal symptoms.
- May reduce the risk of hormone dependent cancers.
- Provides most of the essential amino acids.
- Helps reduce cholesterol
- Low in fat.
- Promotes healthy heart, arteries, blood pressure.

Soy Lecithin:

- **Is an antioxidant which is**

considered a Power Nutrient.

- A natural antioxidant, used by every cell in the body.
- Without lecithin every cell membrane would harden.
- Forms a protective sheath around the brain.
- Protects against arteriosclerosis and heart disease by inhibiting fatty build-up
- Known to promote energy.
- Great in helping to repair a damaged liver due to alcoholism.
- Enables fat to be dispersed in water and removed from the body.
- Vital organs and arteries are protected from fatty build-up.

Soy Protein Isolate:

- Provides most of the essential amino acids.
- No cholesterol.
- Low in fat.
- Has isoflavones which are antioxidants and may help with menopause symptoms.
- May reduce the risk of hormone dependent cancers.
- Provides genistein and daidzein.
- Promotes healthy blood serum cholesterol.

Spearmint:

- Essential oils help relieve fatigue and stress.
- Very good in minerals like potassium that helps control heart rate and blood pressure.
- Rich in antioxidant vitamins A, C and others.

Spinach:

- **Heart smart food**.
- It's one of the best leafy green vegetables you can it. It contains folate, potassium, magnesium, iron and more.
- Rich in vitamin A, C, K, B-complex and folates.
- Prevents some cancers.
- Helps control cholesterol.
- Builds blood.
- Stops bleeding.
- Good for dry skin.
- Used to treat constipation.
- Good for urinary difficulty.
- Rich in iron and chlorophyl.

Spirulina Algae (Whole):

- **Is considered a super food**.
- Spirulina is a blue green algae, considered

to be the most nutrient dense food on earth.

- Unique food source that is an algae with protein concentration 20 times that of soybeans.
- Allergies
- High cholesterol
- Anemia
- Control blood sugar.
- Viral infections.
- Cardiovascular diseases.
- Liver damage
- Inflammatory conditions
- Aids in mineral absorption and cholesterol reduction.
- Curbs appetite.
- Fights cancer by boosting natural killer cells and interferon gamma. Controls abnormal cell growth.
- Boosts the immune system.
- Used to treat malnutrition, anemia, weight loss, and stress.

Stevia:

- Sweet with near-zero calories.
- Many sterols and antioxidants can reduce risk of pancreatic cancer.
- Certain glycosides found to dilate blood vessels, increase sodium excretion and urine output.

- Inhibit cries causing bacteria in the mouth.

Strawberries:

- **Brain booster**.
- Significant amounts of phyto-chemicals that benefit against cancer, aging, inflammation and neurological diseases.
- Excellent source of vitamin C and B-complex.
- Good amount of vitamin A, E and health promoting antioxidants.
- Contain good amount of minerals that help control heart rate, blood pressure, good for bones and teeth.
- Nutritional Facts:
  - Serving Size – 5.3 oz.
  - Calories – 50
  - Fat – 0g
  - Dietary Fiber – 2 g
  - Sugars – 8 g
  - Protein – 1 g

Sucrose:

- Commonly called table sugar.
- Used as a flavoring.
- Used as a sweetener.
- Source of energy.

Suma (Pfaffia Paniculate):

- Brazilian Ginseng.
- Gives the body energy over a sustained period of time rather than short term.
- Tends to calm the body.
- Gives muscle mass and endurance.
- Contains high amounts of the trace element germanium.
- Commonly used for cancer remedies.
- Helps in immune system restoration.
- Enhances the action of oxygen in the body.
- May make one sleepy if you take too much.

Sunflower seed:

- Rich in polyunsaturated fatty acid.
- Also good monounsaturated fatty acid which helps to prevent coronary artery disease and stroke.
- Good source of protein.
- Contain healthy benefiting poly-phenol compounds which help reduce blood sugar levels.
- Rich in vitamin E and B-complex.
- Helps reduce anxiety and neurosis.
- Rich source of essential minerals.
- Nutritional Facts:
    - Serving Size – 1 oz.
    - Calories –165

- Dietary Fiber – 3.1 g
- Protein – 5.5 g

Superoxide Dismutase (S.O.D.):

- **Is an antioxidant which is considered a Power Nutrient.**
- Enzyme which reduces rate of cell destruction.
- Revitalizes cells and destroys free radicals.
- Utilizes minerals in body.
- Slows aging.
- Relieves pain.
- First line of defense against oxygen toxicity.
- Used to treat arthritis and joint disorders.
- Useful in treating side effects of cancer.
- Alleviates prostate problems.
- Useful in treatment of Peyronie's disease.
- Helpful in treatment of Amyotrophic Lateral Sclerosis.

Sweet marjoram:

- Very popular herb, especially in Mediterranean region.
- Contain certain chemicals that have anti-inflammatory and anti-bacterial properties.
- High levels of vitamin C.
- Exceptional high levels of vitamin A which helps protect from lung and oral cavity

cancers.
- Zea-xanthin proven beneficial against age-related macular disease.
- Very rich in vitamin K which limits neuronal damage in the brain.
- Good amounts of minerals like iron, potassium, etc.

Sweet Potatoes:

- Sweet potatoes are packed with added fiber.
- Excellent source of vitamin A, C, K and some B-complex.
- Prevents some cancers.
- Nutritional Facts:
  - Serving Size – 4.6oz.
  - Calories – 100
  - Fat – 0 g
  - Dietary Fiber – 4 g
  - Sugars – 7 g
  - Protein – 2 g

Swiss Chard:

- Many phytonutrients that have health promotional and disease prevention properties.
- Excellent source of vitamin C, K, and A.
- Helps prevent some cancers.

- Helps the body boost immunity.

Tang Kuei:

- Angelica sinensis, commonly known as "dong quai" or "female ginseng" is a herb from the family Apiaceae, indigenous to China.
- Famous herb used to balance female hormones and nourish the female glandular system.
- Particularly effective in treating menstrual cramps and other cyclical symptoms as well as alleviating the discomforts of menopause.
- Powerful blood purifier and antispasmodic.
- Useful against hypertension and anemia.

Tarragon:

- Tarragon used as a traditional remedy to stimulate appetite and alleviate anorexic symptoms.
- Help in lowering blood-glucose levels.
- Helps prevent clot formation in side tiny vessels.
- Rich source of vitamin A, C and others.

Taurine:

- **Is an amino acid and is considered a Power Nutrient**.

- Is a major constituent of the digestive secretion bile.
- Reduced amounts contribute to weight gain.
- It can help reduce blood sugar.
- Can reduce defects in nerve blood flow and motor nerve conduction.
- It can improve nerve function in diabetics.
- Recommended supplementation of 2,000 mg daily for cardiovascular and metabolic support.

Tea:

- **Heart smart food**.
- Major source of antioxidant flavonoids.

Theanine:

- **Is an amino acid and is considered a Power Nutrient**.
- Reduces stress and anxiety without the tranquilizing effects found in other calming agents.
- Stimulates the brain's production of alpha waves, making you feel relaxed but alert.
- Recommended supplementation of 100 to 400 mg daily for calming benefits.

Theobroma Cacao Extract:

- Used as a diuretic.

- Known to dilate blood vessels.
- Works on the nervous system and brain to feel better emotionally.
- Is a mild stimulant.

Thiamine (Vitamin B1):

- Promotes growth.
- Aids digestion, especially of carbohydrates.
- Improves mental attitude.
- Fights against air or sea sickness.
- Helps treat Herpes.
- Fights against Beriberi disease.

Thyme:

- Essential oils found to have antiseptic and anti-fungal characteristics.
- Very high antioxidants levels.
- Rich with vitamin A, C, E, and K.
- Stress relief.

Tocopherols Mixed :

- **Is an antioxidant which is considered a Power Nutrient.**
- Sometimes added to protect flavor.
- Key to cellular respiration.
- Prevents cell damage and repairs tissue while reducing scarring.
- Critical to the normal clotting of the

blood.
- Strengthens capillary walls and produces red blood cells.
- Seems to have a dramatic effect on the reproductive system of both males and females.
- Can be a diuretic to the system.

Tomato:
- **Heart smart food**.
- Helps control cholesterol
- Helps prevent colon, prostate, breast, endometrial, lung, oral cavity and pancreatic cancers.
- High in vitamin A, C and B-complex.
- Nutritional Facts:
    - Serving Size – 5.3oz.
    - Calories – 25
    - Fat – 0 g
    - Dietary Fiber – 1 g
    - Sugars – 3 g
    - Protein – 1 g

Tomato Concentrate (Fruit):
- Useful in preventing Cancer.
- High in Vitamin A & C.
- Source of Potassium which is good for the heart.
- Useful treatment for colds and flu.
- Great for prostate health.

Triglycerides, Medium Chain:

- Medium sized essential fatty acids.
- Useful for athletes.
- Supplies fast source of energy.
- Increases metabolism.
- Helps develop muscles.

Tryptophan:

- **Is an amino acid and is considered a Power Nutrient**.
- It plays a part in wound healing.
- It has the ability to increase levels of serotonin, a calming neuro-transmitter.
- Recommended supplementation of 500 to 4,000 mg daily for insomnia and depression.

Turmeric:

- Source of major antioxidant catechins.
- A member of the Ginger family.
- Also known as Curcuma Longa.
- Adds flavor.
- Improves digestion.
- Stimulates circulation.
- Relaxes spasms.
- Alleviates pain.

- Aids in indigestion, low blood pressure, colic, morning sickness, flu.
- Helpful with neuro generative diseases such as multiple sclerosis.
- Used to treat flatulence, jaundice, menstrual problems, and hemorrhage.
- Inhibits production of inflammation related enzymes which are found in cancers, especially bowel and colon and certain inflammatory diseases.
- Prevents free radical damage.
- Improves rheumatoid arthritis.
- Improves respiratory disorders.

Tyrosine:

- **Is an amino acid and is considered a Power Nutrient**.
- Is synthesized from the amino acid phenylalanine, which is derived from food.
- Useful during conditions of stress, fatigue, work, sleep deprivation, and elevated stress hormone levels.
- Recommended supplementation of 1,000 mg daily for mental and physical enhancement.

Uncaria Tomentosa (Cat's Claw):

- Grown in the Andes Mountains of Peru.
- Oxyindole alkaloids are the active

ingredient that helps stimulate the immune system.
- The alkaloids along with glycosides may be the reason why this herb has an anti-inflammatory and antioxidant action.
- Helps with ulcers, tumors, inflammation, intestinal problems, and arthritis.
- Useful in healing wounds.

Uva Ursi Extract:

- A plant species commonly referred to as bearberry. Found in Europe, Asia and North America.
- Excellent diuretic.
- Good for urinary tract inflammations.
- Dissolves stones.
- Is a blood purifier and stops bleeding.

Valerian (Root):

- A hardy perennial flowering plant, with heads of sweetly scented pink or white flowers. Native to Europe and parts of Asia.
- Well known strong sedative and sleep aid.
- Good for spasms, cramps, and pain in general.
- Improves circulation.
- Reduces mucus.

Vanilla beans:

- The word vanilla, derived from the diminutive of the Spanish word *vaina*, meaning sheath or pod. The vanilla bean is a long thin fruit. Vanilla is the second most expensive spice after saffron.
- Small amounts of B-complex vitamins. Help in enzyme synthesis, nervous system function and regulating body metabolism
- Trace amounts of minerals like potassium.

Vitamin A:

- **Is an antioxidant and is considered a Power Nutrient**.
- Vitamin A can be found in two principal form in foods. Retinol, the form of vitamin A absorbed when eating animal food sources. The carotenes alpha-carotene, beta-carotene, etc. which come from other food sources than animal.
- Slows aging.
- Protection against lung and oral cavity cancers.
- Enhances immunity by protecting mucous membranes.
- Prevents night blindness and other eye problems.
- Great for skin disorders.
- Utilizes protein.
- Key in formulation of bones and teeth.

- Enhances growth and repair of body tissue.

Vitamin B₁ (Thiamin Hydrochloride):

- Vitamin B_1 or Thiamin is a water-soluble vitamin of the B complex.
- It must be obtained from food and therefore is considered an essential nutrient. Grains are the most important dietary sources of thiamine.
- Helper in energy yielding reactions.
- Promotes growth.
- Aids digestion, especially of carbohydrates.
- Improves mental attitude.
- Fights against air or sea sickness.
- Helps treat Herpes.
- Fights against Beriberi disease.

Vitamin B₂ (Riboflavin):

- Vitamin B_2 is also known as Riboflavin. It is found in foods like milk, cheese, leaf vegetables, beans and almonds. It is also available by supplements.
- Necessary for cell formation, reproduction, and growth.
- Maintains good vision, nails, hair, and skin.
- Essential in breakdown of carbohydrates, fats, and proteins.

- Facilitates oxygen use and antibody production.

Vitamin B₃:

- Vitamin B$_3$ is also known as Niacin. Niacin is found in a variety of foods including chicken, fish, peanuts, and beans. It is also available via supplement.
- Helps schizophrenia.
- Lowers cholesterol.
- Promotes healthy skin.
- Aids the nervous system.
- Helps metabolize carbohydrates, fats, and proteins.
- Aids digestion.

Vitamin B5:

- Vitamin B5 is also known as Pantothenic acid. Small quantities are found in most foods. The major source is meat and whole grains are another good source. Vegetables like broccoli and avocados are also a good source.
- Wonderful aid in healing wounds.
- Fights infection.
- Builds antibodies.
- Helps prevent fatigue.
- Reverses toxic effects of many antibodies.
- Good for hypoglycemia, ulcers, and blood and skin disorders.

- Critical to cell metabolism.
- Is activating agent.
- Releases energy from carbohydrates, fats, and proteins.
- Increases production of cortisone, steroids, and antibodies.

Vitamin B 6:

- Vitamin B6 is a water-soluble vitamin part of the B complex group. Several forms of B6 are known.
- Good sources of B6 are meats, whole grain, vegetables, nuts and bananas. It is also available via supplements.
- Involved in more body functions than any other single nutrient.
- Essential to synthesis of RNA, DNA, and, therefore, directly affects the reproduction and growth of all cells.
- Helps in absorption of fats and proteins as well as in the stimulation of proper digestive juices, so is critical in the weight loss process.
- Aids in production of digestive juices.
- Red blood cells coenzyme and antibody formulator.
- Maintains balance of sodium and potassium.
- Insures the smooth functioning of both the immune and nervous systems.
- Necessary for production of hydrochloric

acid.
- Decreases symptoms of P.M.S.
- Helps with allergies, arthritis, and asthma.
- Been known to help carpal tunnel syndrome.
- Helps heart by reducing cholesterol around it.
- Enhances the immune system.
- Aids production of antibodies.

Vitamin B9:

- Vitamin B9 is also known as Folic acid or folate. Folate which is from the Latin word *folium*, mean leaf is found naturally in many foods, and among plants especially plentiful in dark green leafy vegetables.
- Is coenzyme in DNA process of cell division and replication.
- Essential to embryonic and fetal development and prevention of mental retardation.
- Is a carbon carrier, brain food and increases energy.

Vitamin B12:

- Vitamin B12 is also called cobalamin.
- Vitamin B12 is from bacteria in animals and found in most animal derived foods, including fish, poultry, eggs, and dairy. It

is also available in things like kombucha cultured tea and fermented tea that both use bacterial and yeast to create.
- Important in cell formation and longevity.
- Prevents anemia.
- Counters nerve damage and maintains fertility.
- Aids greatly in digestion and absorption process.
- Found to increase energy.
- Helps to restore mental abilities dealing with memory loss and mental clarity.
- Helps to deal with stress.
- Calms irritability.
- Helps prevent diabetic complications.

Vitamin C:

- **Is an antioxidant and is considered a Power Nutrient.**
- Vitamin C is found in many fruits and vegetables. It is also the most widely taken nutritional supplement.
- Greatly enhances immunity as well as adrenal gland function.
- Aids tissue growth and repair.
- Good for bones.
- Prevents hemorrhaging.
- Maintains collagen formation in connective tissue.
- One of the major antioxidants.
- Reduces effects of allergy producing

substances.
- Reduces capillary fragility and enhances it on uptake.
- Recommended supplementation is 1,000 – 2,000 mg daily.

Vitamin D:

- **Vitamin D is considered a Power Nutrient**.
- Vitamin D is a group of fat-soluble vitamin. In humans, the most important compounds in this group are vitamin D3.
- The primary source of vitamin D is sunlight exposure. Small amounts of Vitamin D are also found in some foods. Supplementation is important since people do not always get the daily amount of required sunlight.
- Important for calcium and phosphorus absorption; which is necessary for normal growth and development.
- Helps synthesize the enzymes in the mucous membranes that transport calcium.
- Maintains stable nervous system and normal heart action and blood clotting.
- Prevents rickets and osteoporosis.
- One of the most important nutrients in preventing disease.
- Is a major help in prevention of flu.
- Low D is associated with allergies, arterial

stiffness, asthma, autism, autoimmune disease, breast cancer, cardiovascular disease, chronic fatigue syndrome, colon cancer, decreased cognitive function & mental agility, decreased physical function, depression, hypercholesterolemia, hypertension, immune system dysfunction, insulin resistance, low birth weight, metabolic syndrome, osteoporosis, pancreatic cancer, parkinson's disease, poor blood sugar control, poor muscle strength, pre-eclampsia, rheumatoid arthritis, upper respiratory infections, urinary incontinence in women, weak bones and teeth

- Children whose mothers did not receive enough vitamin D during pregnancy may have: low calcium in neonatal blood, poor postnatal growth, increased incidence of autoimmune diseases later in life

- Recommended supplementation: For flu prevention and overall better health, children need 2,000 IU per day, while adults need 5,000 to 10,000 IU per day. It has also been shown to help overcome the flu if you start this program early. Take 2,000 IU per kilogram of body weight each day for three days.

Vitamin E:

- **Is an antioxidant and is considered a Power Nutrient.**

- Is a powerful fat soluble antioxidant.
- Vitamin E refers to a group of eight fat-soluble compounds. It can be found in corn oil, soybean oil, wheat germ oil, sunflower and safflower oils. Supplements are also suggested.
- Key to cellular respiration.
- Prevents cell damage and repairs tissue while reducing scarring.
- Critical to the normal clotting of the blood.
- Strengthens capillary walls and produces red blood cells.
- Seems to have a dramatic effect on the reproductive system of both males and females.
- Can be a diuretic to the system.
- Seems to reduce coronary heart disease.
- The A-Alpha Tocopherol form has been linked to inflammation reduction.
- Seems to diminish arthritic pain.
- Used in conjunction with Vitamin C in the treatment of cataracts.
- Helps control epileptic seizures.
- Helps cause the disappearance of granuloma annulare, a skin disease.
- Improves glucose tolerance and insulin sensitivity, especially in diabetics.
- Useful in stabilizing patients with chronic skin ulcers.
- Useful in reducing heavy blood flow in females.

- Recommended supplementation: Vitamin E is 800 IU to 1,000 IU per day.

Vitamin H:

- Vitamin H is also known as Biotin and B7 is a water-soluble B vitamin.
- Biotin is found in a variety of foods. Swiss chard and raw egg yolk are high in biotin. However, the consumption of egg whites with egg yolks minimizes the biotin.
- Good for cell growth and fatty acid production.
- Helps in metabolism of carbohydrates, fats, proteins, and the B complex vitamins.
- Important to healthy bone marrow and nerve tissue.
- Stimulates sweat glands and normal skin and hair.
- Is coenzyme in DNA process of cell division and replication.
- Essential to embryonic and fetal development and prevention of mental retardation.
- Is a carbon carrier, brain food and increases energy.

Vitamin K:

- Vitamin K is a group of fat-soluble vitamins. They come from a number of vegetable sources like Spinach, Broccoli,

Swiss Chard and lettuce.
- Necessary for blood clotting.
- Helps maintain bone mass.
- A catalyze in the prevention of osteoporosis.
- Help limiting neuronal damage in the brain.
- Established role in treatment of Alzheimer's disease.
- Used as an anticoagulant.

Walnut:

- Rich in monounsaturated fatty acids to help prevent coronary artery disease and strokes.
- Good in omega-3 fatty acids. Anti-inflammatory action lower the risk of blood pressure, coronary artery disease, strokes and breast, colon and prostate cancers.
- Rich in phyto-chemical substances which have potential health effects against cancer, aging, inflammation and neurological diseases.
- Excellent source of vitamin E.
- Rich in many minerals. Help with digestion and nucleic acid syntheses.
- Nutritional Facts:
  - Serving Size – 1 oz.
  - Calories –185
  - Dietary Fiber – 1.9 g

– Protein – 4.3 g

Walnut, Black (Leaf):

- Using the leaf as a tea has been useful in lowering blood sugar, cleansing the blood, and eliminating intestinal parasites.
- In tea form useful as an astringent.
- The leaves seem to have an antibiotic element.
- The bark as well as the leaves can be useful in the treatment of skin troubles such as herpes, eczema, or indolent ulcers.
- Works well on diarrhea, constipation, and dysentery.
- Acts as an antifungal and may help in yeast infection.
- Useful in de-worming and eliminating parasites.
- Helps in toning the GI tract.
- Helpful in balancing the intestinal flora.
- Useful in helping with the absorption of oil-soluble vitamins including Vitamin B12 in association with ileocecal inflammations.

Watercress:

- Good source of vitamin A, C, K and B-complex.
- Helps prevent some cancers.

- Helps in treatment of Alzheimer's.
- Helps with regulation of the heart.

Watermelon:

- Excellent source of vitamin A which protect from lung and oral cavity cancers.
- Rich in antioxidants that protect cells and other structures.
- Excellent source of lycopene that protects skin from UV rays.
- Good source of potassium that protects against stroke and coronary heart diseases.
- Nutritional Facts:
  - Serving Size – 10.0 oz.
  - Calories – 80
  - Fat – 0g
  - Dietary Fiber – 1 g
  - Sugars – 20 g
  - Protein – 1 g

Wheatgrass:

- **Is considered a super food**.
- Regulates normal cell growth.
- Power detoxifier protects the liver and the blood, and neutralizes toxic substances.
- Blood builder – the chlorophyll in wheatgrass is almost identical in chemical composition to hemoglobin, the compound that carries oxygen in the

blood.

Whey:

- High source of amino acids from cow's milk that can be utilized by the body for fuel
- Helps maintain muscle mass.
- Contains little or no lactose
- Whey consists of three types: whey protein isolate, whey protein concentrate, and hydrolyzed whey protein.

Whey Protein:

- Dairy based source of amino acids.
- Contains the amino acid leucine that inhibits the atrophy of muscles after a trauma or during severe stress.
- Contains branched-chain amino acids like leucine and valine which aid people with Lou Gehrig 's Disease and with liver disease as well as intense exercise.
- The product that remains after the removal of fat and casein from milk.
- Used in food processing to texturize, process and add nutrition.

Wild Lettuce:

- Contains amino acids, minerals, and vitamins.
- Useful for insomnia because of lactucin.

- Useful in alleviating restlessness and excitability (especially in children).
- Used for dysmennhorea.
- Used for coughs.
- Improves circulation, decreases cholesterol.
- Helps to reduce blood sugar.
- Contains carminative properties which help with flatulence and bloating.

Yams:

- Good source of vitamin A, C and B-complex.
- Helps prevent some cancers.

Yerba Maté Extract:

- Yerba Maté begins as a shrub and then matures to a tree that grows up to 15 meters. It is grown in northern Argentina.
- Enhances healing power of other herbs.
- Good for allergies, blood purifier.
- Appetite controller and diuretic.
- Stimulates production of cortisone and helps depression, fatigue and stress.
- The plant contains 24 vitamins and minerals, 15 amino acids, potent antioxidants.
- Stimulates the body without nervous side effects.

Zeaxanthin:

- Zeaxanthin is one of the most common carotenoid alcohols found in nature. It is the pigment that gives paprika, corn saffron and other plants heir characteristic color.
- Useful in decreasing risk of macular degeneration.
- Helps protect retina from damaging effects of light.
- May lessen brain damage due to stroke.
- Helpful with cancer.
- Useful with atherosclerosis.
- May be helpful with prostate cancer.
- Helpful in preventing and treating breast cancer.
- Helpful in eliminating skin cancer from UV rays.
- Decreases inflammatory process involved in the lung disease COPD (chronic obstructive pulmonary disease).

Zinc:

- Zinc is an essential mineral of exceptional biologic and public health important. Zinc deficiency affects over two billion people in the developing world and is associated with many diseases.
- Zinc is included in most multi vitamin

supplements. Preparations include zinc oxide, zinc acetate and zinc gluconate.
- Considered to be assimilated easier than other forms of zinc.
- Each have their own importance to the body.

Zinc Amino Acid Chelate:

- Critical to the body in small amounts.
- Important in the synthesis of nucleic acid, RNA & DNA.
- Essential to the normal functioning of the reproductive organs, particularly to the prostate and sperm production.
- Used for centuries to speed the healing of wounds both internally and externally.
- Enhances taste bud acuity.
- A component of insulin.
- Protects liver from damage.
- Helps skin disorders.
- Critical to protein synthesis.
- Aids digestion, absorption and metabolism of vitamins.
- Important in collagen formation and immune system functioning.
- Recommended supplementation is 15 to 30 mg daily.

Zinc Gluconate:

- Is one of the major antioxidants.
- Critical to the body in small amounts.
- Aids digestion, absorption and metabolism of vitamins.
- Important in collagen formation and immune system functioning.

Zinc Oxide:

- Critical to the body in small amounts.
- Important in the synthesis of nucleic acid, RNA & DNA.
- Essential to the normal functioning of the reproductive organs, particularly to the prostate and sperm production.
- Used for centuries to speed the healing of wounds both internally and externally.
- Enhances taste bud acuity.
- A component of insulin.
- Protects liver from damage.
- Helps skin disorders.
- Critical to protein synthesis.
- Aids digestion, absorption and metabolism of vitamins.
- Important in collagen formation and immune system functioning.

Zucchini:

- Good source vitamin C, B-complex and

folates.
- Antioxidants to help with health.

Illnesses Reference

(Our research shows that the suggested nutrients may be helpful with the following*)

Optimal Health and Preventative Health Care

- A balanced diet
- Exercise
- Sleep
- Water
- Positive thinking
- Vitamins and Minerals
- Essential Fatty Acids
- Antioxidants
- Healthy Proteins
- Healthy Fats
- Fruits and Vegetables.

Acid Reflux:
- (see digestive)

Addictions:

- Kudzu + Antioxidants + Omega 3 Fish Oil
- Blood Cleansing and Liver Repair
- B Complex
- Calcium
- Magnesium
- Vitamin C

- Bioflavonoids
- Niacin
- Ginseng
- Valerian
- Jujube Extract
- Ashwagandha Extract
- Soy Lecithin
- L-Glutamine
- Cysteine

ADHD:
- Omega −3

Aging:
- (see optimal health)
- Acai
- Argine
- Dark chocolate
- Mulberries
- Pumpkin

Allergies:
- Aloe Vera
- Bee Pollen
- Calcium
- Magnesium
- Multi-Vitamins
- Vitamin C
- Antioxidants
- Vegetase

- Protease
- Quercetin

Anemia:

- (see energy)

Anxiety:

- (see stress)

Arthritis:

- (see inflammation)

Asthma:

- (see respiratory & Allergies)

Athletic Muscle Building:

- Proteins
- Medium Chain Triglycerides
- L-Argllline
- L-Carnitine
- Hydrochloride
- Vitamins A & C
- Argine
- Lysine

Athletic energy and endurance:

- Carbohydrates
- Multi- Vitamins & Minerals

- Guarana
- Green Tea
- Inositol
- Chromium
- Thiamin Hydrochloride
- Caffeine
- Astragalus
- Licorice
- Ginseng
- Glycine
- Nettle
- Oats
- Sea Buckthorn
- L-Glutamine.
- Maca

Athletic Recovery:
- (combating free radical damage due to strenuous exercise)
- Protectors from Free Radical Damage.
- A Variety of Antioxidants.
- Nitric Oxide a precursor to L-Arginine
- Alpha Lipoic Acid
- Lysine

Bone/Skeletal:
- (helpful with: osteoporosis, broken bones, bone growth, and related bone

health)
- Calcium
- Magnesium
- Soy
- Vitamin A
- Vitamin C
- Vitamin D
- Vitamin K
- Boron
- Folic Acid
- Black Cohosh
- Horsetail
- Glucosamine
- Copper
- Silicon Dioxide
- Hesperidin
- Beta Caro
- Omega – 3
- Basil
- Dark chocolate
- Pomegranate

Brain:

- (preventing or postponing problems with: Alzheimer's disease memory dementia)
- Omega 3 Fish Oil –
- Coenzyme Q10
- Alpha-Lipoic Acid

- Lecithin
- Multiple Vitamin & Minerals
- Pycnogenol
- Grape Seed Extract
- L-Arginine
- Watercress
- Asparagus
- Brussels sprouts
- Camu – Camu
- Caraway
- Cilantro
- Cucumber

Bronchitis:

- (see Respiratory & Immune)

Cancer:

- (helpful with: all types of cancers tumors and some studies show that some of these may alleviate some of the effects of radiation and chemotherapy)
- Reishi Mushroom
- Pycnogenol
- Shiitake
- Bilberry
- Quercetin
- Green Tea
- Pomegranate
- Astragalus

- Vitamins A C & E
- Rosemary
- Schizandra
- Lycopene
- Lutein
- Fiber
- Aloe Vera
- Protease
- Vegetase
- Omega 3 Fish Oil - HLL
- Garlic
- Turmeric
- Calcium
- Magnesium
- Alpha-Lipoic Acid
- EPA
- Arugula
- Asparagus
- Avocado
- Basil
- Borage
- Brussels sprouts
- Butternut squash
- Brazil nuts
- Cantaloupe
- Caraway
- Carrot
- Chia seed
- Cilantro
- Collard greens
- Dates

- Flax seed
- Hazelnut
- Kale
- Kiwi
- Lemon
- Mango
- Moringa
- Mulberries
- Mustard
- Okra
- Olive
- Papaya
- Peach
- Pecan
- Pineapple
- Pistachio nuts
- Plums
- Quinoa
- Radishes
- Rhubarb
- Spinach
- Sweet potato
- Swiss chard
- Tomato
- Walnut
- Watermelon
- Yams

Capillary Fragility:

- Rutin

- Vitamin C

Candida:

- (see detox)
- Acidophilus
- Aloe Vera
- Essential Fatty Acids
- Garlic
- Quercetin
- Calcium
- Magnesium
- Vitamins A C D & E.
- Multivitamin and Minerals
- B-Complex
- Coenzyme Q-10
- Beta-Carotene
- Bioflavonoid
- Pycnogenol
- Protease
- Vegetase
- Lycopene
- Cranberry
- Schizandra
- Dark chocolate

Cardiovascular

- (see circulatory)

Cataracts:
- (see eye)

Cholesterol:
- Artichoke
- Avocado
- Burdock root
- Jalapeno peppers
- Leeks
- Oats
- Pear
- Salmon
- Spinach
- Tomato

Circulatory:
- (helpful with: diabetes cold hands/feet)
- L-Arginine
- L-Camitine
- L-Citrulline
- Coenzyme Q-10
- Cayenne
- B Complex
- Vitamin C
- Vitamin A
- Calcium
- Niacin
- Pycnogenol
- Grape Seed Extract

- Cleansing Herbs
- Omega 3 Fish Oil – HLL
- Garlic
- Potassium
- Argine
- Banana
- Pomegranate
- Sesame seeds
- Tarragon
- Walnut
- Watermelon

Cirrhosis of the Liver:

- (see Alcohol and Detox)

Colds:

- (see Immune)

Constipation:

- (see Digestive)

Cramps:

- Calcium
- Valerian
- Tang Kuei
- Multi Vitamin and Mineral Supplements

Crohn's Disease:

- B-complex
- omega 3
- Krill Oil
- Vitamin K
- Vegetase
- Protease
- Garlic
- Lactobacillus
- L- Glutamine
- Aloe

Dental:

- (helpful with: bleeding gums, cavities, gingivitis, periodontal disease)
- Aloe Vera
- Vitamin C
- Bioflavonoids
- Multi-Vitamin
- Quercetin
- Coenzyme Q-10
- Vitamin A C and E
- Rosemary
- Goldenseal
- Friendly Bacteria
- Zinc
- Grape Skin Extract
- Allsice

Depression:

- Melatonin
- Niacin
- Omega 3 Fish Oil - HLL
- Fish Oils
- Krill Oil
- Green Tea
- English Lavender
- Buckwheat

Detox / Cleanse:

(helpful with: liver damage, air, water, and food pollutants, heavy metals, and allergies)

- Aloe Vera
- Apple Pectin
- Dandelion
- Fructooligosaccharides
- Grapefruit Bioflavonoids
- Hesperidin
- Lactobacillus Acidophilus
- Cat's Claw
- Garlic
- Barberry Root
- Black Walnut Leaves
- Bromelain
- Castor Oil
- Catalase
- Fenugreek
- Goldenseal
- Buckthorn

- Lemon Oil.
- Wheatgrass

Diabetes:

(helpful with: type I and type II, hypoglycemia, hyperglycemia & insulin resistance)
- Chromium
- Fiber
- CoQ10
- Protein
- Omega-3 Fish Oil - HLL
- Clove Oil
- Vitamin and Mineral Supplements
- Alpha-Lipoic Acid
- Krill oil
- Bilberry
- Cloves
- Schizandra
- Wild Lettuce
- Gymnema Sylvestre
- Garcinia Cambogia
- Riboflavin
- Argine
- Pantothenic Acid
- Beans and legumes
- Chia seed
- Mulberries
- Olive
- Pomegranate

- Taurine

Diarrhea:

- (see Digestive)

Digestive / Gastrointestinal Tract:

(help with: Crohn's, indigestion, acid reflux, constipation, diarrhea, ulcers, hemorrhoids.)

- Proteases
- Fiber
- Friendly Bacteria
- Vegetase
- Aloe
- Orange Peel
- Krill Oil
- Nettle
- L-Glutamine
- Asparagus
- Banana
- Caraway
- Carrot
- Coriander seeds
- Horseradish
- Oregano
- Peppermint
- Pineapple
- Plums
- Spinach
- Taurine

Dysentery:

- (see Digestive)

Ear:

- Carrot

Energy:

(helpful with: anemia, fatigue, chronic fatigue syndrome, tiredness, and exhaustion)

- Bilberry
- Beta-Carotene
- Vitamin A
- B-Complex
- Vitamin C
- Vitamin E
- Zinc
- Calcium
- Selenium
- Copper
- Manganese
- Bioflavonoids
- Turmeric
- Lutein
- Zeaxanthin
- L-Arginine
- L-Citrulline
- Olive Oil

- Beta Carotene.

Epilepsy:
- Niacin
- B Complex
- Folic Acid
- Magnesium
- Calcium Zinc
- Coenzyme Q-10
- Melatonin
- Vitamins A C & E
- L-Arginine
- Alpha-Lipoic Acid
- Black Cohosh
- Aloe Vera
- Schizandra
- Rosemary
- Omega 3 Fish Oil- HLL.

Eye:
(helpful with: glaucoma, macular degeneration, cataracts, blurred vision, vascular retinopathy, color blindness, general eye care)

- Bilberry
- Beta-Carotene
- Vitamin A
- B-Complex
- Vitamin C
- Vitamin E

- Zinc
- Calcium
- Selenium
- Copper
- Manganese
- Bioflavonoids
- Turmeric
- Lutein
- Zeaxanthin
- L-Arginine
- L-Citrulline
- Olive Oil
- Beta Carotene
- Alpha-Lipoic Acid
- Basil
- Butternut squash
- Camu – Camu
- Cashew nut
- Dark chocolate
- Dates
- Kale

Fibromyalgia Syndrome:

(Help with: chronic fatigue syndrome)

- Alpha-Lipoic Acid
- Astragalus
- B Complex
- Coenzyme Q-10
- Bioflavonoids
- Black Walnut Leaf:

- Calcium
- Magnesium
- Fibers
- Friendly Bacteria
- Garlic
- Grape Skin Extract
- L-Arginine
- L-Camitine
- L-Citrulline
- Lecithin
- Omega 3 Fish Oil - HLL
- Olive Leaf
- Potassium

Food Poisoning:

(helpful with: botulism, Campylobacter infection, salmonellosis, staphylococcal, etc.)

- Aloe Vera
- Acidophilus
- Bioflavonoids
- Fructooligosaccharides
- Garlic
- Goldenseal
- Milk Thistle
- Omega 3 Fish Oil- HLL
- Red Clover
- Rosemary
- Schizandra
- Vitamins A C & E.

Flu:

- (see Immune)

Free Radical Damage:

- (see Oxidative Damage)

Fungus:

- (see Candida)

Gastrointestinal Tract:

- (See Digestive)

Gout:

- Turmeric
- Garlic
- Milk Thistle
- Omega-3 Fish Oil - HLL
- Fish
- B Complex
- Vitamin C
- Bioflavonoids
- Potassium
- Superoxide Dismutase
- Zinc
- Calcium
- Glucosamine

Hay Fever:
- (see allergies)

Heartburn:
- Aloe Vera
- Protease
- Vegetase

Heart Disease:

(helpful with: aneurysm, arrhythmia, atherosclerosis, cardiomyopathy, congestive heart failure, high blood pressure, angina, high cholesterol, high triglycerides, high homocysteine, heart attack)
- Coenzyme Q-10
- Vitamins A E & C
- Calcium
- Magnesium
- Fiber
- Friendly Bacteria
- Alpha-Lipoic Acid
- Garlic
- L-Arginine
- L-Carnitine
- L-Citrulline
- Lecithin
- Choline
- Green tea
- Omega 3 Fish Oil - HLL

- Fish
- Krill Oil
- Olive Leaf
- Potassium
- Selenium
- Superoxide Dismutase
- Melatonin
- Multiple Vitamins
- Phytosterol Ester
- Pomegranate
- Argine
- Banana
- Basil
- Bay leaf
- Beans and legumes
- Buckwheat
- Burdock root
- Butternut squash
- Brazil nuts
- Cantaloupe
- Caraway
- Cardamom
- Cashew nut
- Cherry
- Chia seed
- Chili pepper
- Cucumber
- Dark chocolate
- Dates
- Dill
- Hazelnut

- Kiwi
- Macadamia nuts
- Olive
- Peach
- Pecans
- Resveratrol
- Sesame seeds
- Watermelon

Hepatitis:

- Proteins
- Protease
- Acidophilus
- Soy
- Whey
- Milk Thistle
- Coenzyme Q-10
- Superoxide Dismutase
- Vitamins A C & E
- Bioflavonoids
- Garlic
- Dandelion Leaf
- Goldenseal
- Green Tea
- Calcium
- Magnesium
- Wheatgrass

Immune:

(helpful with: lupus, cancer, colds, flu,

herpes)

- **Vitamin D is essential**
- Reishi Mushroom
- Pycnogenol
- CoQ10
- Shiitake
- Bilberry
- Quercetin
- Green Tea
- Astragalus
- Vitamins A C & E
- Rosemary
- Schizandra
- Lycopene
- Lutein
- Fiber
- Aloe Vera
- Protease
- Vegetase
- Omega 3 Fish Oil- HLL
- Krill Oil
- Garlic
- Turmeric
- Calcium
- Magnesium
- Alpha-Lipoic Acid.
- Argine
- Cysteine
- Dark chocolate
- Lemon
- Lysine

- Okra
- Oregano
- Papaya
- Quinoa
- Swiss chard

Indigestion:

- (see Digestive)

Infertility:

- (see Reproductive)

Inflammatory:

(helpful with: arthritis, Crohn's, bursitis, gout, lupus, rheumatism, osteoarthritis)

- Nettle
- Bromelain
- Uncaria Tomentosa (Cat's Claw)
- Glucosamine
- Pantothenic Acid
- Omega 3 Fish Oil - HLL
- Fish Oil
- Krill Oil
- Superoxide Dismutase
- Vitamins A C & E
- Bioflavonoids
- Calcium
- Garlic
- Melatonin

- Orange Fruit Bioflavonoids
- Quercetin
- Basil
- Olive
- Pineapple

Injuries (healing time):

- Argine

Insomnia:

- (see Sleep)

Irritable Bowel Syndrome:

- (see Digestive)

Joint:

(helpful with: cartilage joints)
- Olive Oil
- Omega 3 Fish Oil - HLL
- Orange Bioflavonoids
- Protease
- Bioperine
- Boswellia
- Endopeptidase
- Glucosamine Sulfate
- Methylsufonylmethane
- Clove Oil
- Tumeric

- Vitamins A C & E
- Carrot Extract
- Cranberry Extract
- Ashwagandha Extract
- Eleutherococcus
- Krill Oil
- Argine
- Camu – Camu
- Carrot

Liver:
- (see Hepatitis Cirrhosis)

Lupus:
- (see Inflammation)

Mental Health:
- Omega – 3
- Maca

Migraine:
- (see Pain)

Menopause:
(helpful with: hot flashes,   night sweats, irritability, insomnia, dry vagina, low libido, bladder problems, heart palpitations)
- Lecithin

- Cinnamon Bark
- Vitamins A C & E
- Bioflavonoids
- Black Cohosh Extract
- Calcium
- Kudzu Extract
- Red Clover Extract
- Soy Extract
- Protease
- Omega 3 Fish Oil - HLL
- Vegetase
- Multivitamin & Mineral Supplements
- Magnesium
- L-Arginine
- Zinc
- Potassium
- Selenium
- Krill Oil
- Oregano

Metabolic Syndrome:
- Alpha-Lipoic Acid
- CoQ10
- Green tea
- Pomegranate

Nervous system:
- (see Stress)

Oxidative Damage Free Radical Damage:

- Vitamin A C & E
- Alpha-Lipoic Acid
- Lutein
- Zeaxanthin
- Rosemary
- Schizandra
- Lycopene
- Sea Buckthorn
- Milk Thistle
- Melatonin.

Pain:

(helpful with: joint   muscular   headaches
  migraine)

- Valerian
- Ashwagandha
- Hops Extract
- Passion Flower
- Cinnamon Bark
- Nettle
- Magnesium Taurate.
- Cardamom seed
- Dark chocolate

Parasites:

- (see detox)

PMS (Premenstrual Syndrome:

(helpful with: bloating, anxiety, backache, cramps, irritability, depression, headaches, fatigue, and insomnia.)

- Melatonin
- Acidophilus
- Calcium
- Magnesium
- Pantothenic Acid
- B Complex
- Vitamins A C D & E
- Beta-Carotene
- Bioflavonoids
- Zinc
- Lecithin
- Omega 3 Fish Oil- HLL
- Choline
- Inositol
- Milk Thistle
- Black Cohosh
- Ashwagandha Extract
- Passion Flower
- Krill Oil.
- Dark chocolate
- Maca
- Oregano

Prostate:

- Lycopene
- Saw Palmetto

- Pumpkin Seed Oil
- Selenium
- Soy Lecithin
- Vitamin E
- Coenzyme Q-10
- Superoxide Dismutase
- Vitamin A
- Beta-Carotene
- Vitamin C
- Bioflavonoids
- Garlic
- Acidophilus
- Dandelion
- Red Clover
- Buchu
- Goldenseal
- Omega 3 Fish Oil – HLL
- Pumpkin seed

Psoriasis:

- Milk Thistle
- Protease
- Multiple Vitamin and Mineral Supplements
- Omega 3 Fish Oil- HLL
- Carotene
- Zinc
- Vitamins A C D & E
- Lecithin
- Selenium

- Aloe Vera
- Soy Whey
- Krill Oil

Reproduction:

(help with: infertility, erectile dysfunction, impotence, low libido)

- L-Giutamine
- L-Arginine
- L-Citrulline
- Vitamin E
- Ginseng
- Eleuthero Extract
- Glycine
- L-Arginine
- Aspartic Acid
- Pycnogenol
- Iron.
- Argine
- Maca

Respiratory:

- Zeaxanthin
- Eleutherococcus Extract.
- Camu – Camu

Sleep:

(helpful with: insomnia and sleep disorders)

- Calcium

- Amla Fruit
- Cinnamon Bark
- English Lavender
- Hops Extract
- Wild Lettuce
- Orange Peel
- Passion Flower
- Valerian Root
- Melatonin
- Magnesium
- Pumpkin

Stress:

(helpful with: Anxiety, Irritability (see depression), muscular pains (see pain), ulcers (see digestive), Heart (see Heart)).

- Sleep
- Exercise
- Good Friends
- Spontaneous Fun
- Multiple Vitamin & Mineral Supplements
- Calcium
- B Complex
- Vitamin A C & E
- Antioxidants
- L-Arginine
- Schizandra
- Rosemary
- Krill Oil

- Alpha-Lipoic Acid
- Calcium
- Magnesium
- English Lavender
- Wild Lettuce Leaves
- Melatonin.
- Banana
- Cherry
- Maca
- Quinoa
- Sesame seeds
- Sunflower seed
- Theanine
- Tryptophan
- Tyrosine

Sunburn:

- Aloe Vera
- Alpha-Lipoic Acid
- Antioxidants
- Bioflavonoids
- Calcium /
- Magnesium
- Lutein
- Lycopene
- Potassium
- Quercetin
- Rosemary
- Vitamin A
- Carotenoids

- Vitamins C & E
- Zinc
- Horsetail
- Omega 3 Fish Oil –HLL
- Krill Oil.

Thyroid, Hypo (Too Little):

- Kelp
- Bilberry
- Calcium
- Dandelion
- Milk Thistle
- Magnesium
- Iodine
- Vitamin A Carotenoids
- Vitamin C Bioflavonoids
- Omega 3 Fish Oil - HLL
- Chromium
- Protease
- Krill Oil

Ulcers, Stomach:

- Aloe Vera
- Pectin
- Acidophilus
- Apple Pectin
- Chamomile
- Vitamin E
- Vegetase
- Uncaria Tomentosa

- Omega 3 Fish Oil - HLL
- Curcuma Longa (Tumeric)
- Pycnogenol
- Spinach
- Vitamin A
- Carotenoids
- Vitamin C
- Bioflavonoids
- Vitamin K
- Zinc
- Multivitamin

Urinary / Bladder:

(helpful with: bladder and urinary infections and disorders.)

- Alliin
- Bilberry
- Blueberry
- Calcium
- Cranberry
- Bioflavonoids
- Nettle Garlic
- Vitamin C
- Water.

Weight Loss:

(helpful with: overweight obesity)

- Soy
- Medium Chain Triglycerides

- L-Arginine
- L-Citrulline
- Whey
- Chromium
- Fiber
- Protein
- CoQ10
- Omega 3 Fish Oil - HLL
- Clove Oil
- Vitamin & Mineral Supplements
- Alpha-Lipoic Acid
- Bilberry
- Cloves
- Pomegranate
- Schizandra
- Wild Lettuce
- Garcinia
- Krill Oil
- Argine
- Beans and legumes
- Cucumber
- Pear
- Pine nuts

Weight Gain:

(helpful with: small or weak muscles anorexia underweight)

- Protease
- Fiber
- Friendly Bacteria

- Absorption and Assimilation Ingredients
- Vegetase
- Aloe
- Orange Peel
- Krill Oil
- Endopeptidase
- Nettle
- Proteins
- Soy
- Whey
- Medium Chain Triglycerides
- Omega 3 Fish Oil - HLL
- Calcium
- Nutritious Calories
- Vitamins A C and E
- Green tea

Worms:

- (see detox)

(* These statements have not been evaluated by the Food and Drug Administration. Although a nutrient may be shown to help one person with a particular illness; it does not mean it will help all people. These statements are not intended as prescriptions or cures.)

ABOUT THE AUTHOR AND MORE FOR YOU

Rod Stone *is the principle partner of* ***Rod Stone Group*** *and they focus on providing information on health, nutrition, and many other subjects to improve your life.*

I began writing articles on health and nutrition in the mid '90s. In 2004 I started full time working with people and providing information and products to assist with health and nutrition. In 2008 I started to become involved with the importance of specialized high intensity workouts. In 2011 we became involved in Universal Energy and related fields.

Our nutritional and product site @ http://herbal-nutrition.net/rodstone has products and information on Weight Management, Fitness and Energy, Immune Solutions, Stress Management, Digestive Health, Women's Health, Men's Health, Children's Health, Healthy Aging and Sports Nutrition.

We have written dozens of books and hundreds of articles. We also have hundreds of websites to help people improve their life. You can find the links to these at: http://rodstonegroup.com/.

Find out the books available on Amazon by checking the author central area for Rod at: http://www.amazon.com/Rod-

Stone/e/B001KCWDXE/ref=sr_ntt_srch_lnk_2?qid=1
384817706&sr=1-2

WE HAVE A SPECIAL FOR YOU!!!

At our media store we have over a thousand different books, audio and video products for your benefit. We keep all of these at a huge discount of over 70% all the time. **We have an extra special for those that buy this book. Go to our media store at http://www.rodsmediastore.com/ and when you sign in you can send us a message with subject "Amazon" and our support staff will send you a reply and from then on all of your purchases will be at 50% off our sale prices. That means that an items that retails for $10, you can get for less than $1.50**

We also have great products to improve your life including many free ones at http://rsmediagrp.com/free-books/.

We believe that "information is today's currency."

To your success,
Rod Stone Group

www.ingramcontent.com/pod-product-compliance
Lightning Source LLC
Chambersburg PA
CBHW060452290526
45791CB00001B/87